W9-DES-394

Surgical Pathology Dissection

Gene M. Fino, M.D.
1996

Springer

New York
Berlin
Heidelberg
Barcelona
Budapest
Hong Kong
London
Milan
Paris
Santa Clara
Singapore
Tokyo

Surgical Pathology Dissection

An Illustrated Guide

Ralph H. Hruban, M.D.
Department of Pathology
The Johns Hopkins University
School of Medicine
Baltimore, MD

William H. Westra, M.D.
Department of Pathology
The Johns Hopkins University
School of Medicine
Baltimore, MD

Timothy H. Phelps, M.S.
Department of Art as Applied to Medicine
The Johns Hopkins University
School of Medicine
Baltimore, MD

Christina Isacson, M.D.
Department of Pathology
The Johns Hopkins University
School of Medicine
Baltimore, MD

With a Foreword by Frederic B. Askin, M.D.

 Springer

Ralph H. Hruban, M.D.
Department of Pathology
Meyer 7-181
The Johns Hopkins Hospital
600 North Wolfe Street
Baltimore, MD 21287-6971, USA

William H. Westra, M.D.
Department of Pathology
Meyer 7-181
The Johns Hopkins Hospital
600 North Wolfe Street
Baltimore, MD 21287-6971, USA

Timothy H. Phelps, M.S.
Department of Art as Applied to Medicine
The Johns Hopkins University
School of Medicine
1830 East Monument Street, Suite 7000
Baltimore, MD 21205-2100, USA

Christina Isacson, M.D.
Department of Pathology
Pathology 709
The Johns Hopkins Hospital
600 North Wolfe Street
Baltimore, MD 21287-6971, USA

Cover illustration: Pancreaticoduodenectomy for cancer of the pancreas. A single section can be taken to demonstrate the relationship of the carcinoma to the pancreas, to the bile duct, to the ampulla of Vater, and to the duodenum. Illustration by Timothy H. Phelps.

With 50 Illustrations

Library of Congress Cataloging-in-Publication Data
Surgical pathology dissection : an illustrated guide / Ralph H.
    Hruban . . . et al. ; foreword by Frederic B. Askin.
        p. cm.
    Includes bibliographical references.
    ISBN 0-387-94567-9 (alk. paper)
    1. Pathology, Surgical—Laboratory manuals.   2. Human dissection-
-Laboratory manuals.   I. Hruban, Ralph H.
    [DNLM: 1. Pathology, Surgical—laboratory manuals.
    2. Dissection—laboratory manuals.   WO 142 S9615   1995]
    RD57.S87 1995
617'.07—dc20
DNLM/DLC
for Library of Congress   95-24467

Printed on acid-free paper.

Production managed by Terry Kornak; manufacturing supervised by Jacqui Ashri.
Typeset by Bytheway Typesetting Services, Inc., Norwich, NY.
Printed and bound by R.R. Donnelly & Sons, Willard, OH.
Printed in the United States of America.

9 8 7 6 5 4 3 2 1

ISBN 0-387-94567-9   Springer-Verlag New York Berlin Heidelberg

To the Breakfast Club. Fond memories of hooping it up.

To my wonderful wife, Claire, and our three terrific children, Zoe, Emily, and Carolyn

Ralph H. Hruban

To Mike, brother and friend

William H. Westra

To my wife Lyn, for her ever present love and support; my two children, Katie and Kevin, who bring me great and constant joy; to my art instructors of the past for all they have shared with me; and particularly and most importantly, my Father; and in loving memory of my Mother

Timothy H. Phelps

To my parents for all their love and encouragement

Christina Isacson

Foreword

The modern surgical pathology cutting room is replete with tools of the electronic age. Computers, automatic cassette labelers, bar coding, and even electronic voice-recognition systems are available to help the surgical pathologist be an effective, efficient, and highly productive cog in the machinery of health care delivery. In spite of this automated armamentarium, much of our ability to render diagnoses rests with the surgical pathology "cutters." These personnel need to be trained to handle surgical specimens consistently and appropriately, with the goal of providing optimal diagnostic information and adequate pathologic correlation with clinical and radiologic findings.

This dissection manual is an outgrowth of what Waldemar Schmidt has called the "oral tradition" of surgical pathology. Traditionally, the senior pathologist passed down to the trainee an individual accumulation of expertise on the handling of specimens. This transfer of information was often random and based solely on the specific case at hand. Now, despite the importance of training personnel, the exigencies of modern practice limit the amount of time available for individual training, and so most laboratories have developed their own local manual. Unfortunately, many of these manuals are incomplete or not user-friendly.

Drs. Hruban, Westra, and Isacson have prepared this manual with the help of a distinguished and talented medical artist. Tim Phelps's pen and ink drawings bring a unique vitality and multidimensional effect to the reader throughout the manual as dissection techniques are explained and illustrated. The editors and contributors have effectively shared their talents and experience by providing general principles that can be employed to resolve even the most complex problems in dissection and effective tissue sampling. The methods are broadly applicable and unusually easy to follow.

This text should be at hand in all surgical pathology laboratories, where it will be useful to a wide variety of personnel including staff pathologists, residents, pathologist's assistants, histotechnologists, and other laboratory personnel. It is highly likely that many surgeons would also benefit from use of this manual, through which they can gain an understanding of how specimens are dissected and can become familiar with the way in which margin and tumor sampling are carried out.

This is a very practical manual. The authors discuss the clinically important features of various types of specimens and lesions in each organ system. They instruct the prosector in every instance as to what information is needed to provide the clearest clinical picture. I suspect that this work will be most valuable to the surgical pathology cutter late in the evening or on weekends, when the redoubtable oral historian of surgical pathology is not available. This manual should serve as a cornerstone on which to build a stable but malleable standard of excellence in the surgical pathology cutting room.

Frederic B. Askin, M.D.
Professor of Pathology
The Johns Hopkins University
School of Medicine
and
Director of Surgical Pathology
The Johns Hopkins Hospital
Baltimore, MD 21287-6971, USA

Preface

Our goal in writing this book is to provide an illustrated, hands-on guide for the dissection of surgical pathology specimens. It is intended for use by anyone involved in the gross evaluation and handling of surgical tissues, whether they be technicians, pathologist's assistants, medical students, residents, or staff pathologists. Several outstanding dissection manuals, such as Schmidt's *Principles and Techniques of Surgical Pathology* (1983), provide a comprehensive approach to the evaluation of pathology specimens, but their practical utility in the daily hustle and bustle of a laboratory can be limited. It is our impression that there is a need for an illustrated manual that provides a logical and concise approach to the most commonly encountered specimens.

This guide begins with an overview of how to approach any surgical pathology specimen and follows with a description of laboratory techniques and photography. The remainder of the manual is arranged by organ system. All ranges of specimen types are described, from biopsies to total resections. Each chapter includes a description and illustration of the mechanics involved in handling a specimen as well as a conceptual framework for questions to keep in mind during the dissection. At the end of each chapter, the section entitled "Important Issues to Address in Your Surgical Pathology Report" includes most of the information needed to provide accurate TNM (the International Union Against Cancer's Clinical Stage Classification of Malignant Tumors) and FIGO (Fédération Internationale de Gynécologie et d'Obstetrique) staging for the majority of tumors. The reader may choose to read this manual straight through in its entirety; however, the chapters can also be read selectively, as dictated by the type of specimen encountered. The illustrations are intended to stand on their own and can be easily displayed at the work station. We hope that this illustrated guide will make the dissection of any specimen an informative and enjoyable endeavor.

Ralph H. Hruban, M.D.
William H. Westra, M.D.
Timothy H. Phelps, MS
Christina Isacson, M.D.

Acknowledgments

The authors thank Amanda Lietman for her superb assistance in preparing, proofreading, and editing this manual and for her patience and understanding. It is impossible to praise her talents and efforts enough. The authors also thank Drs. Frederic B. Askin and Grover M. Hutchins for their constructive criticism of the book and Drs. Michael Borowitz, David Eisele, Jonathan Epstein, Kristin Fiebelkorn, Stanley R. Hamilton, Zdenek Hruban, Wayne Koch, Ralph Kuncl, Robert Kurman, and Charles Yeo for sharing their expertise. The authors also thank Jane Day, Claire E. Hruban, and Cheryl Dewyre.

Contents

I. General Approach and Techniques

II. The Head and Neck

III. The Digestive System

IV. The Cardiovascular/Respiratory System

V.   Bone, Soft Tissue, and Skin

VI.   The Breast

VII.   The Female Genital System

VIII.   The Urinary Tract and Male Genital System

IX.   The Ocular System

X.   The Endocrine System

XI.   Pediatric Tumors

XII.   The Central Nervous System

XIII.   The Hematopoietic and Lymphatic System

XIV.   Odds and Ends

Contributors

Frederic B. Askin, M.D.
Professor of Pathology, The Johns Hopkins University School of Medicine; and Director of Surgical Pathology, The Johns Hopkins Hospital, Baltimore, MD 21287-6971, USA

Norman J. Barker, M.S., R.B.P.
Assistant Professor of Pathology and Art as Applied to Medicine; and Assistant Director of Pathology Photography, The Johns Hopkins University School of Medicine, Baltimore, MD 21287-6971, USA

Peter C. Burger, M.D.
Professor of Pathology, Oncology, and Neurosurgery, The Johns Hopkins University School of Medicine, Baltimore, MD 21287-6971, USA

William M. Fox, III, B.S., M.S.
Pathologist Assistant, The Johns Hopkins Hospital, Baltimore, MD 21287-6971, USA

W. Richard Green, M.D.
International Order of Odd Fellows Professor of Ophthalmology; and Professor of Pathology, the Wilmer Ophthalmological Institute, The Johns Hopkins University School of Medicine, Baltimore, MD 21287-6971, USA

Thomas D. Horn, M.D.
Associate Professor of Dermatology and Pathology, The Johns Hopkins University School of Medicine; and Director of Dermatopathology, The Johns Hopkins Hospital, Baltimore, MD 21287-6971, USA

Ralph H. Hruban, M.D.
Associate Professor of Pathology and Oncology, The Johns Hopkins University School of Medicine; Assistant Professor of Otolaryngology, Head and Neck Surgery, The Johns Hopkins University School of Medicine; and Director, Division of Cardiovascular-Respiratory Pathology, The Johns Hopkins Hospital, Baltimore, MD 21287-6971, USA

Christina Isacson, M.D.
Fellow in Gynecologic Pathology, The Johns Hopkins University School of Medicine, Baltimore, MD 21287-6971, USA

Edward F. McCarthy, Jr., M.D.
Associate Professor of Pathology and Orthopedic Surgery, The Johns Hopkins University School of Medicine; and Director, Bone Histomorphometry Laboratory, The Johns Hopkins Hospital, Baltimore, MD 21287-6971, USA

Elizabeth J. Perlman, M.D.
Assistant Professor of Pathology, The Johns Hopkins University School of Medicine; and Director, Division of Pediatric Pathology, The Johns Hopkins Hospital, Baltimore, MD 21287-6971, USA

Timothy H. Phelps, M.S., FAMI, C.M.I.
Associate Professor of Art as Applied to Medicine, The Johns Hopkins University School of Medicine, Baltimore, MD 21287-6971, USA

Robert H. Rosa, Jr., M.D.
Fellow in Ophthalmic Pathology, The Wilmer Ophthalmological Institute, The Johns Hopkins University School of Medicine, Baltimore, MD 21287-6971, USA

William H. Westra, M.D.
Assistant Professor of Pathology, The Johns Hopkins University School of Medicine, Baltimore, MD 21287-6971, USA

I General Approach and Techniques

1 General Approach to Surgical Pathology Specimens

Safety in the Surgical Pathology Laboratory

The key to safety in the surgical pathology laboratory is to recognize that this area is a dangerous place. A variety of noxious chemicals are routinely used in the surgical pathology laboratory, and tissues infected with the human immunodeficiency virus (HIV), hepatitis viruses, mycobacteria, and other agents enter through its doors on a daily basis. Not only are these infectious agents present in the laboratory, but their transmission is also facilitated by the frequent handling of bloody tissues and the routine use of surgical blades, knives, saws, and other sharp instruments. Clearly, the surgical pathology laboratory is no place to "let down one's guard" by becoming careless or distracted. Rather, safety in the work area should become an ingrained habit, and universal precautions should be exercised with all specimens.

Protective Gear

The prosector should regard all tissues as potentially infectious, not just those tissues removed from patients known to have an infectious disease. For the protection of oneself and for the safety of others, the prosector should wear protective gear in the cutting area at all times. Protective gear prevents contact of potentially infectious materials with the skin and mucous membranes, and it diminishes the transfer of infectious material outside of the surgical pathology laboratory. At the very least, protective gear should include a scrub suit, waterproof shoe coverings, a surgical gown and/or waterproof forearm wraps, gloves, a cap, a mask, and eye protection. A waterproof apron should also be worn to prevent the absorption of fluids onto the clothing and skin. Hands should be protected by well-fitting surgical gloves. To prevent seepage of fluids, two pairs of gloves are preferred to one pair, and these gloves should be changed frequently. Keep in mind that even two pairs of gloves will not protect against punctures and cuts. Fine mesh metallic or synthetic gloves that are cut-resistant are recommended in those instances where one is unfamiliar with the use of a sharp instrument or when one is dissecting a specimen with sharp edges (e.g., a bone resection). Soiled or bloody garments and coverings should not be worn outside of the cutting area.

Disposal of Instruments and Trash, and Storage of Specimens

In order to avoid inadvertent wounds, there should be no more than one blade in the dissection field at any one time. Needles, razor blades, scalpel blades, and other sharp disposable objects should be promptly discarded into appropriate containers following their use. Trash items soiled with blood or other potentially infectious materials should be discarded into designated biohazard containers located in the cutting area. Upon completion of the dissection, the specimen should be stored in a container with adequate formalin. Specimen containers should be wiped clean of any potentially infectious materials, securely closed to prevent leakage, accurately labeled, and stored in a designated storage area. In cases of known viral hepatitis, HIV infection, or tuberculosis, the cutting area should be washed clean and wiped with a disinfectant such as dilute bleach, and a biohazard label should be affixed to the specimen container.

Fundamentals of Dissection

At first glance the challenges facing the surgical pathology cutter appear almost insurmountable. The types of specimens that come across the cutting table seem endlessly diverse, and the complexity of these specimens may at times be confounding. To top it off, each specimen, whether a simple needle biopsy or a convoluted composite resection, must be handled with equal care and precision. How then does one confidently and effectively function in the surgical pathology laboratory, given the bewildering diversity and complexity of specimens that enter its doors? Where does one even begin?

For any specimen, the best place to begin is at the end. Even before making the first cut, take time to visualize the end result of your work, the surgical pathology report. Consider the issues that need to be addressed in that report, and then plan a dissection of the specimen that will help address these important issues. While it is true that no two specimens are exactly alike, you will find that the questions they pose are remarkably similar. Even the most complex of specimens can be reduced to three fundamental issues: *What structures are present? What is the nature of the pathologic process? How extensive is that process?* Regardless of the complexity or novelty of the specimen, these issues can be efficiently addressed by conforming the dissection to a systematic four-step approach. By mastering these four fundamental steps of surgical dissection, the surgical pathology cutter will be well equipped to tackle even the most intimidating of specimens with confidence.

Step 1. Specimen Orientation

If the surgical pathology report is the end result of the dissection, specimen orientation might be regarded as a road map by which to reach that ultimate destination. With orientation, an otherwise confusing conglomerate of tissue is placed in its proper clinical and anatomic context and appreciated as a structural unit. Then a proper course of dissection can be chartered. Without orientation, specimen dissection can proceed speedily but may never reach its desired aims.

The Requisition Form

Orientation is usually thought of in terms of the structural anatomy of the specimen. While these anatomic considerations certainly are important, a specimen must also be understood in terms of its clinical context. No specimen should be dissected in a "clinical vacuum"; rather, a strategy for the dissection of any specimen should be directed by the clinical history. For example, a uterus removed for leiomyomas is handled very differently from one removed for cervical cancer. Fortunately, clinical orientation usually does not require a full review of the patient's medical chart. Instead, a pertinent clinical history can often be succinctly communicated through a requisition form (Appendix 1-A). The requisition form should accompany every surgical specimen. It identifies the patient and the type of specimen, provides relevant clinical history, and alerts the prosector to specific biohazards. Sometimes the information on the requisition form may not be complete, or a case may be so complex that additional clinical information is required. These situations may necessitate a review of the medical chart, evaluation of imaging studies, and/or direct communication with the requesting clinician. Do not be shy or timid; if in doubt, call the clinician.

Anatomic Orientation

The anatomic orientation is best appreciated at the outset of the dissection while the specimen is still intact. The further the dissection progresses, the more difficult it can become to reconstruct and orient the specimen. Even when the specimen is entirely intact, orientation is not always a simple task. Unlike the surgeon viewing the specimen as it is situated in the patient, the prosector frequently cannot fully appreciate the anatomic context of the isolated specimen lying on the cutting table. Nonetheless, two steps can be taken to overcome this obstacle and confidently orient the specimen: *appreciation of anatomic landmarks* and *communication with the surgeon*.

Anatomic landmarks can be thought of as consistent features (a shape, a contour, a structure, etc.) that serve to indicate a specific structure or designate a position. For example, the uterus can be correctly oriented by the relative positions of its peritoneal reflections, and the orientation of the eye may be guided by the insertion of a specific extraocular muscle. Before proceeding with any dissection, the prosector should be familiar with the anatomy of a specimen and should be able to recognize and interpret its unique anatomic landmarks. Toward this end, an anatomy atlas should be within easy reach of the cutting table.

Sometimes, even with the guidance of an anatomy atlas, the prosector may not be able to orient the specimen. Either the specimen is too complex, or it simply does not possess any useful anatomic landmarks. In these instances, communication with the surgeon takes on a very important role. This communication may take one of several forms. Sometimes a surgeon will use tags, sutures, and/or an accompanying diagram to designate important structures or locations on a specimen. At other times, specimen orientation may require direct communication with the surgeon.

Step 2. Dissecting the Specimen

The Cutting Station

The cutting station should be clean and orderly. Most routine dissections require a ruler, a scale, a scalpel with disposable blades, scissors, forceps, a probe, and a long sectioning knife. At the beginning of each day, the prosector should make certain that these tools are well maintained, clean, and within easy reach. Between dissections, these instruments and the cutting table itself should be rinsed clean of fluids and tissue fragments. This practice will help eliminate contamination of a specimen with tissue fragments from a prior dissection. Similarly, sectioning blades should be rinsed regularly during a dissection so that fragments of a friable tumor are not inadvertently transferred throughout the specimen.

No more than a single specimen should be on the cutting table at any one time. Although it may seem time efficient to work on multiple specimens simultaneously, this dangerous practice openly invites the loss and mislabeling of specimens. For example, a small biopsy is easily overlooked and discarded when overshadowed by a large and messy specimen on the same cutting table, while specimens of similar size and shape may easily be confused and mislabeled.

Handling of Tissues

While all tissues are to be handled cautiously and gently, small specimens in particular are susceptible to ill-treatment. Small and delicate tissue fragments may be crushed during transfer to a tissue cassette, they may desiccate if not placed in fixative in a timely manner, and they even may be lost during processing if they are not easily seen. These problems can be minimized by adhering to a few simple guidelines:

1. Small specimens should never be forcibly squeezed between the ends of a forceps or the tips of the fingers. Instead, small specimens should be gently lifted from the specimen container using the end of a wooden applicator stick or pickups. Alternatively, small specimens can be filtered directly into a tissue bag, avoiding instrumentation altogether.

2. Small specimens should be quickly placed in fixative. Ideally, most small specimens (i.e., less than 1 cm) should reach the surgical pathology laboratory already in fixative. This requires that physician offices, biopsy suites, and operating rooms be supplied with appropriate fixatives, and that all personnel involved be instructed as to their proper use. Sometimes delays in fixation are necessary, as when a frozen section is required or when special tissue processing is indicated. In these instances, the tissue should be kept damp in saline-soaked gauze. Never leave small tissue fragments exposed to the air on the cutting table, and never place these small fragments directly on a dry paper towel. These practices are sure to hasten tissue desiccation.

3. For extremely small specimens, the journey from specimen container to histologic slide is a treacherous one, and they may be lost at any point along the way. For this reason, it is a wise practice to identify these small tissue fragments first and then mark the fragments so that they can be found more easily by the histotechnologist. Before the specimen container is even opened, check its contents for the size and number of tissue fragments, and record these in the gross description. If no tissue is seen or if inconsistencies with the requisition form are noted, carefully open the lid and thoroughly examine the surfaces of the specimen container (including the undersurface of the lid) for adherent tissue fragments. If no tissue is found or if discrepancies persist, the submitting physician should be notified immediately, and the outcome of this investigation should be documented in the gross description.

Once all of the tissue is identified in the specimen container, efforts should be taken to ensure that it safely reaches the histology laboratory and that it is easily identified for embedding and sectioning. Minute tissue fragments should be wrapped in porous paper or layered between porous foam pads before they are placed in the tissue cassette. Before these fragments are submitted to the histology laboratory, they can be marked with eosin or mercurochrome so that they are easier for the histotechnologist to see.

Inking the Specimen

Various inks and colored powders can be used to mark critical points on the specimen. These dyes and powders may help orient both the gross specimen and the histologic section. For example, colored tattoo powder sprinkled on the outer surface of a cystic cavity can be used to distinguish between the outer and inner aspects of the cavity. Similarly, India ink can be painted on the surgical margins so that they can be easily recognized at the time of histologic examination. Indeed, many times the critical distinction of whether or not a neoplasm extends to the surgical margin entirely depends on the absence or presence of ink.

Given the important implications of an inked surface, these dyes should be carefully and judiciously applied to the gross specimen. Keep in mind that just as the effective use of dyes can facilitate the histologic interpretation, the careless and improper use of these dyes can befuddle the microscopic findings. Consider, for example, the implications of sloppily applied ink that runs across a surface where it does not belong. The following guidelines outline the proper application of dyes:

• If possible, apply ink before sectioning the specimen.
• Do not use excessive ink.
• Dry the surface of the specimen with paper towels before applying ink. When applied to a dry surface, ink is more likely to stick to the desired surface and less likely to run onto other areas of the specimen.
• Allow the ink to dry before further processing the specimen. Do not cut across wet ink, as the knife is likely to carry the ink onto the cut surface.

Opening and Sectioning the Specimen

The manner of opening and dissecting specimens is variable, depending on the type of specimen and the nature of the lesion. Bone marrow biopsies may simply be placed directly into a tissue cassette without any further manipulation, while the dissection of complex bone resections may require a multistep process involving special chemical reagents, imaging machines, and bone saws. Although this manual provides specific dissection guidelines for most of the specimens you will encounter, a few general guidelines underlie many of the instructions.

First, localize the lesion before opening the specimen. One effective way to localize the lesion is simply to palpate the specimen. For example, a small peripheral lung tumor may be readily appreciated simply by palpating the lung parenchyma, and a colorectal tumor can usually be detected by probing the lumen of the specimen with a gloved finger. Sometimes further measures are needed to localize the lesion. Review of specimen radiographs, for example, may be necessary to uncover the size and location of a lesion when it involves a bone. Once the lesion is localized, the specimen can be opened in the plane that best demonstrates the pathology.

Second, open the specimen in such a way as to expose the lesion while maintaining its relationships to surrounding structures. In general, the walls of hollow structures (e.g., large bronchi, stomach, intestines, etc.) should be opened along the side opposite the lesion to maintain the structural integrity of the lesion and to preserve important anatomic relationships. For tumors involving solid organs, the specimen should be cut along the longest axis of the tumor to demonstrate the tumor's greatest surface area.

Third, remember to dissect and examine the entire specimen. Often, the dissection is so focused on a localized lesion that the rest of the specimen is not examined. Incomplete dissections represent lost opportunities to fully disclose the extent of a lesion and to uncover unsuspected pathologic processes.

Fixing the Specimen

Before tissue is processed in the histology laboratory, it should be well fixed. Some institutions prefer to fix the specimen before it is dissected and sampled, while other institutions would rather you dissect and sample the specimen in the fresh state. Each method has its advantages and disadvantages. Specimen fixation greatly facilitates tissue sectioning. For example, tissue fixation permits thin sectioning of fatty tissues, and it helps to preserve the structural detail of thin-walled cysts, mucosal-lined organs, and friable tumors. The major disadvantage of specimen fixation is simply that it takes time. Fixation of larger specimens may require submersion in formalin for a full day or longer. Delays caused by fixation can be eliminated by dissecting and sampling the specimen while it is fresh. Although this practice may compromise the quality of the histologic sections, it can significantly reduce case turnaround time. Thus, the decision to fix or not to fix must strike a balance between optimal histology and timely reports. Most of the dissection descriptions in this manual include a step for fixation. Simply skip this step if your institution does not fix specimens before dissection.

Even when one chooses to fix a specimen, a limited dissection of the fresh specimen is usually necessary. Fixative will not diffuse into the center of an unopened specimen, especially if the specimen is large and fatty. To overcome this, hollow organs and large cysts should be opened and solid tissues should be sectioned. Furthermore, a limited dissection is usually needed to expose a lesion if fresh tissue is required for frozen section evaluation, ancillary diagnostic studies (e.g., cytogenetic studies, flow cytometry, etc.), research purposes, or storage in a tissue bank. These important decisions regarding the distribution of tissue must be made while the specimen is fresh, not after the specimen has been submerged in fixative. A detailed description of the various fixatives available and their uses is given in Chapter 2.

Storing the Specimen

The tissue remaining after a specimen has been thoroughly dissected and sampled should not be discarded. Instead, it should be stored in such a way as to ensure easy retrieval and reconstruction of the specimen. Tissues for storage should be placed in a well-sealed container that holds enough fixative to cover the specimen. For a given case, separate parts should be stored in separate containers. Each container should be clearly labeled with the surgical pathology number, the part number, the patient's name, the patient's medical record number, and a biohazard warning when indicated. Specimens that may be of special interest, either from a teaching, diagnostic, or medicolegal perspective, should be so indicated and stored in a permanent storage area. Medical devices likewise should be placed in a properly labeled container and segregated into an area where they can be stored for long periods of time and easily retrieved. Unlike routine tissue specimens, storage of these prosthetic devices does not require fixation.

When preparing a specimen for storage, anticipate the need to return to the specimen at a later time, either to review the gross findings or to submit more sections for histology. Although the specimen may be quite fragmented and distorted following its dissection, efforts should be taken to reconstruct the specimen before placing it on a storage shelf. There are many examples of how this can be done. Lymph nodes and their associated soft tissues can be separately wrapped and labeled according to their respective regional levels. Residual slices of a serially sectioned organ can be fastened together in their original positions. Important landmarks can be designated with tags or safety pins. These simple methods of reconstructing the specimen can become invaluable later, when, for example, the prosector has to return to a colectomy to find more lymph nodes, to a prostatectomy to submit additional slices of prostate tissue, or to a mastectomy to sample a specific quadrant of the breast.

Step 3. The Gross Description

Correlation between the macroscopic and microscopic findings is important when evaluating a specimen and rendering a diagnosis. Just as glass slides represent a permanent record of the histologic findings, the gross description represents a permanent record of the specimen's macroscopic features. The goal of the gross description is threefold. First, it serves as a descriptive report that enables the reader to reconstruct the specimen mentally and envision the location, extent, and appearance of the pathologic process. Second, it serves as a slide index, enabling the pathologist to correlate each slide to a precise location on the specimen. Third, it accounts for the distribution of the tissue, documenting how a specimen has been apportioned for various diagnostic and research purposes.

To help reconstruct an image of a specimen, the gross description must be logical, factual, and succinct. A logical description is one that follows an orderly sequence. The first sentence should tell the reader what the specimen is and what structures are present. The description should then move from one individual component of the specimen to another in a methodical progression. Proceed from overall to specific, from abnormal to normal, and from relevant to ancillary. The best way to avoid a description that is fragmented and chaotic is to dictate after the specimen has been dissected and examined. This approach allows one to gather all of the information, then integrate the gross findings into a narrative that is comprehensive and complete.

A factual description is one that records the objective characteristics of the specimen. With few exceptions, these characteristics include the size, weight, color, shape, and consistency of the specimen and any specific lesions. Among these, size is particularly important. For example, in resections of neoplasms, the size of the neoplasm is critical in staging the tumor, and the distance from the edge of the tumor to the surgical margin may help to determine the adequacy of excision and the need for adjuvant therapy. For excisions of parathyroid glands, the important distinction between a normal and proliferative gland is made on the basis of the gland's weight.

Quite commonly, the gross description is so diluted by trivial details and technical minutiae that the important macroscopic features are not easily recognized by the reader. A concise dictation is one that ignores this minutiae and records only information that serves to achieve the three goals of the gross description. A leaner description can often be achieved by cutting the fat from two areas of the gross description. First, eliminate verbose descriptions of normal anatomy. Descriptions of normal structures should be restricted to pertinent negative findings, and to terse statements about size, color, consistency, and shape that help reconstruct the appearance of the specimen. Second, do not describe the mechanics of the dissection. These technical details are already laid out in the dissection manual and do not belong in the gross dictation unless they clarify the histologic findings or unless your dissection deviates from routine methods (e.g., inflation of a lung with formalin).

Another important function of the gross description is its role as a slide index (Appendix 1-B). The slide index places each histologic slide in its appropriate anatomic context. Consider, for example, the importance of knowing whether a section of a neoplasm was sampled from the center of a tumor or from the margin of surgical resection. Only the prosector knows for sure where and how the specimen was sampled, and it is the prosector's responsibility to communicate this information in the gross description. This information should be summarized at the end of the gross description in the form of a slide index. The slide index should state the number of pieces submitted in each tissue block, the designations used to identify each tissue block, and the precise meanings of these designations. Tissue designation should strive for simplicity, rationality, and standardization. The designations themselves should use as few letters or numbers as possible, but the meanings of these designations should be specific. For example, two sections of tumor could be designated "TA" and "TB," respectively. Remember that slides are frequently sent to other hospitals for consultation, and so these designations also need to be clear to someone not familiar with your institutional idiosyncrasies.

Finally, the gross description should document the distribution of tissue for diagnostic and/or research purposes. Sometimes tissue may be sent for ancillary diagnostic studies including electron microscopy, cytogenetics, and flow cytometry. In some instances fresh tissue may be frozen and stored in a tissue bank so that it can be retrieved at a later time, or tissue may be requested by various laboratories for research purposes. Not only is it important to supervise (under the guidance of a pathologist) the distribution of these tissues, but it is also important to document in the gross description where the tissue has been sent and for what purposes.

Other methods may be used to supplement the description of the macroscopic findings. Among these, photography (see Chapter 3) plays an especially versatile role. Color photographs help re-create the visual image of the gross specimen. These photographs provide a visual record of the gross findings and can be used for teaching purposes at various conferences and in the classroom. Polaroid photographs can be very helpful in clarifying the slide index. As the specimen is sampled for histologic evaluation, the sampling sites can be indicated directly on the Polaroid photograph (using a water-resistant marker). Liberal photography is a practice that is to be encouraged as an effective supplement to the gross description.

Step 4. Specimen Sampling

Mindless sampling of a specimen introduces errors at two different extremes. At one extreme, tissue sampling is inadequate, either because the number of sections is too few or the quality of sections is too poor. In these instances, important issues cannot be adequately addressed in the surgical pathology report. Forgetting to assess a surgical margin, failing to determine the extent of local tumor infiltration, and neglecting to check for metastases to regional lymph nodes are common examples of inadequate sampling. At the other extreme, tissue sampling can be excessive. An inordinate number of tissue sections may exact a costly toll on the resources of the surgical pathology laboratory.

The key to an approach that is both economical and thorough is *selective sampling*. Selective sampling is a strategic approach which attempts to maximize the information that can be obtained from a given tissue section. As opposed to random and indiscriminant sampling of a specimen, tissue sampling that is selective increases the information that can be obtained histologically, and it requires fewer sections to do so. Appendix 1-C lists some fundamental guidelines for selective tissue sampling.

Sampling a Tumor

The goals of tumor sampling go beyond the question of "What is it?" Tumor sampling is concerned not just with the type of a tumor but also with its histologic grade and the degree to which it has extended into surrounding structures. A tumor should be sampled with the objective of addressing all three of these issues.

In general, most sections of a tumor should be obtained from its periphery. This peripheral zone is often the best preserved region of a tumor, while the central zone is frequently so necrotic that it yields no useful histologic information. In addition, the tumor's periphery demonstrates the interface of the tumor with adjacent tissues. This interface zone may provide evidence regarding where a tumor has arisen (e.g., colorectal carcinoma arising in a pre-existing villous adenoma); important clues about the biologic behavior of the tumor (e.g., capsular invasion of a follicular thyroid carcinoma); and information regarding the degree of local tumor invasion (e.g., depth of invasion into the wall of the colon).

Questions frequently arise regarding the number of sections that should be taken of a tumor. Unfortunately, there is no single answer, since the appropriate number of sections depends on the type of specimen. For example, a single section from a solitary liver nodule may be sufficient to confirm that it is a metastasis,

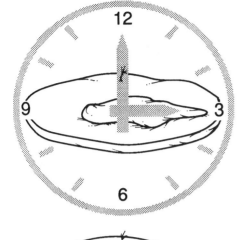

Fundamentals of Specimen Dissection

1. Orient
Use anatomic landmarks and/or surgical designations to help orient the specimen. In the illustration, the surgeon has placed a suture at the 12-o'clock position of the skin ellipse.

2. Measure
Size is one of the most important parameters to document in the gross dictation. Include not only the overall dimensions of the specimen but also the size of the lesion and its distance from the surgical margin.

3. Ink
Application of ink to the cut surface of the specimen is a good way to mark the resection margin.

4. Sample
Adequately sample the specimen. Include sections of the lesion, normal tissue, and the margins. Sections should be no bigger than the diameter and thickness of a nickel.

5. Assess Margins
A perpendicular section is a good way to evaluate the margin when it is closely approached by a lesion. This section shows the distance of the lesion to the edge of the specimen. A parallel section evaluates a larger surface area of the margin, and it may be used to evaluate a margin that is not closely approached by the lesion.

but such limited sectioning of a solitary thyroid nodule may not allow distinction between a follicular adenoma and a follicular carcinoma. Despite this tremendous variability between specimens, a few general considerations should guide the sampling of a tumor. First, when trying to assess the histologic type and grade of a neoplasm, be sure to sample all areas of the tumor that, on gross inspection, appear different. Even strict adherence to rigid rules such as "one section per 1 cm of tumor" may not be adequate if the sections are not selectively taken from areas of the tumor that appear grossly distinct. Second, sections of large cysts should be taken from areas where the cyst wall appears thickened or where the cyst lining has a complex appearance (e.g., shaggy, papillary excrescences, etc). Sections from these areas are most likely to reveal the proliferative areas of the cyst lining and to demonstrate tumor infiltration of the cyst wall. Third, when concern exists about malignant transformation within a benign lesion or premalignant process, the lesion should be extensively if not entirely submitted for histologic evaluation. A number of examples fall under this category, including mucinous cystadenomas of the ovary and pancreas, adenomas of the gastrointestinal tract, Barrett's esophagus with dysplasia, *in situ* transitional carcinoma of the urinary bladder, and many others.

Sampling a Margin

The margin is the edge or the boundary of the specimen. It represents the plane where the surgeon has sectioned across tissues to remove the specimen from the patient. The surgical margin may be free of disease; that is, a rim of uninvolved tissues may surround a pathologic lesion that has been completely resected. Alternatively, the lesion could extend to the edge of the specimen, implying that the lesion has not been completely removed. Clearly, the status of a surgical margin is an important indicator of the potential for the disease to recur and of the need for further therapy. Therefore, the assessment of these margins, both grossly and microscopically, is of considerable importance.

As illustrated, margins can be sampled in one of two ways: They can be taken as either a perpendicular section or a parallel section. A perpendicular section is one taken at a right angle to the edge of the specimen. In this type of section, the true margin is present at one of the two ends of the section. The advantage of a perpendicular section is that it can be used to demonstrate the relationship of the edge of the tumor to the margin. A perpendicular section allows the important distinction between a lesion that truly extends to the margin and a lesion that very closely approaches but does not involve the margin. Since only a small surface area of the margin is represented in a perpendicular section, the margin must be carefully inspected and then selectively sampled from those areas where it is most closely approached by the tumor.

A shave section is one taken parallel to the edge of the specimen. Because the entire shave section spans the margin, a relatively large surface area at the margin can be evaluated with a single section. A shave section is ideal for obtaining complete cross sections of small luminal or cylindrical structures. Unlike the perpendicular section, the shave section does not effectively demonstrate the relationship between the margin and the edge of the tumor. Its major drawback is that it cannot be used to distinguish between a lesion that truly extends to the margin and one that very closely approaches but does not actually involve the margin. For this reason, shave sections should be reserved for those instances when the margin appears widely free of tumor or when dealing with small luminal or cylindrical structures that are not easily sampled using perpendicular sections.

To help the pathologist interpret the histologic findings, the slide index portion of the gross description should clearly document how the margin was sampled. The presence of tumor in a margin section may have entirely different implications, depending on whether the margin was sampled using a perpendicular or parallel section.

Sampling Lymph Nodes

A specimen dissection is not complete until the lymph nodes, when present, have been found and sampled. Sampling of lymph nodes is especially important for resections of neoplasms where critical staging information may depend on the number and location of lymph nodes involved by metastatic tumor.

Although the lymph node status is clearly important in staging neoplasms, finding these lymph nodes can be a tedious and frustrating job. They may be small, inconspicuous, and entirely overshadowed by the fibroadipose tissues in which they are embedded. Skill at finding lymph nodes develops over time, but a few guidelines may enhance the efficiency of your search. First, it is generally best to orient the specimen, designate the various regional lymph node levels, and submit margins of the soft tissues before a lymph node dissection is undertaken. Keep in mind that lymph node dissections require significant distortion and manipulation of the soft tissues such that the specimen may not be easily reconstructed following a thorough search for lymph nodes. Second, many prefer to look for lymph nodes in the fresh specimen. Lymph nodes are often best appreciated by touch, and smaller lymph nodes may elude detection when the surrounding soft tissues have been hardened by fixation.

Lymph nodes larger than 1 cm should be bivalved to allow fixation of the entire node. A common error is to submit both halves of more than one lymph node in the same tissue cassette for histologic evaluation. This may cause considerable confusion regarding the number of involved lymph nodes if more than one tissue fragment contains metastatic tumor. To avoid this confusion, a given cassette should contain the two halves of only one lymph node. Alternatively, the tissue cassette may contain several nodes when only one half of each node is submitted. When submitting only one half of a lymph node, remember to submit the half that looks most abnormal.

Sampling Normal Tissues

Even tissues that do not appear to be involved by a pathologic process should be sampled for histologic evaluation. Histologic evaluation can uncover diseases that may not have been appreciated on gross inspection. These microscopic alterations may be entirely unrelated to the primary lesion, or they may be closely associated findings that provide important insight into the origin of the primary lesion. It is also important to sample normal tissues to document the structures that were surgically removed. For example, a section taken from the adrenal gland in a radical nephrectomy specimen clearly documents that this organ was removed, identified, and examined.

The Surgical Pathology Report

The surgical pathology report is a comprehensive statement that integrates the macroscopic and microscopic findings. It represents the summation of efforts on the part of the prosector, the histotechnologist, and the pathologist. Forms are now available that have standardized the reporting of the pathologic findings in a comprehensive way. For the prosector facing a complex and intimidating specimen, the time to contemplate the content of the surgical pathology report is not after the dissection is completed, but before the first cut is even made. With this in mind, this manual describes the dissections of various specimens, including a tabulation of important issues to address in the surgical pathology report. These lists are provided so relevant clinical issues can be kept in mind as specimens are dissected, described, and sampled.

Appendix 1-A. Information to Be Included in the Specimen Requisition Form

Patient Identification	Type of Specimen	Clinical History	Additional Notations
Full name	Date of specimen collection	Pertinent clinical history	Special requests
Identifying number	Site of specimen	Differential diagnosis	Biohazard alerts
Date of birth	Type of procedure	Operative findings	Name/phone number of physicians to contact

Appendix 1-B. Example: Slide Index for a Modified Radical Mastectomy

Designation	Meaning	No. of Pieces of Tissue
FSC	Frozen section control	1
TA	Tumor—(A = first tissue block)	1
TB	Tumor—(B = second tissue block)	1
UIA	Upper inner quadrant	1
UIB		1
UOA	Upper outer quadrant	1
UOB		1
LIA	Lower inner quadrant	1
LIB		1
LOA	Lower outer quadrant	1
LOB		1
N	Nipple	2
S	Skin	1
LNIA	Level I lymph nodes	3
LNIB		2
LNIIA	Level II lymph nodes	2
LNIIB		4
LNIIIA	Level III lymph nodes	3
LNIIIB		4

Total blocks: 19

Total pieces of tissue: 32

Appendix 1-C. Selective Specimen Sampling

Tumor Sampling

- Sections from the periphery of a tumor are usually more informative than are sections from the center of a tumor.
- For heterogeneous tumors, sample all components of the tumor.
- For cystic lesions, sample areas of the cyst wall that are thickened or lined by a complex surface.
- If there is concern about a hidden focus of malignant transformation within a benign neoplasm or premalignant process (e.g., infiltrating carcinoma arising in a pre-existing villous adenoma), the lesion should be extensively, or even entirely, sampled for histologic evaluation.

Margin Sampling

- Always sample the specimen margins, even from lesions that are clinically felt to be benign (e.g., gastric ulcers).
- Perpendicular sections show the relationship of the lesion to the margin. Perpendicular sections are usually preferred to parallel sections, especially when the margin is closely approached by the tumor.

- Shave (i.e., parallel) sections are sometimes best when the margin appears widely free of tumor or for samples of a cylindrical or tubular structure (e.g., optic nerve or ureter margins).

Lymph Node Sampling for Tumor Staging

- Orient the specimen, submit soft tissue margins, and designate regional lymph node levels before dissecting the soft tissues for lymph nodes.
- Lymph nodes are easiest to find in unfixed tissues where they can be more readily appreciated by palpation.
- Lymph nodes larger than 1 cm should be sectioned to facilitate tissue fixation.
- If a lymph node is sectioned, remember to examine the sections for focal abnormalities.
- Never submit multiple sections from more than one lymph node in a single tissue cassette.

Normal Tissue Sampling

- At least one representative section should be taken from each grossly normal structural component of the specimen.

2 Laboratory Techniques

William M. Fox, III, M.S.
Robert H. Rosa, Jr., M.D.

General Comments

The modern surgical pathology laboratory is equipped to perform a staggering number of routine and special diagnostic procedures. Most are carried out by the laboratory technologist; however, gross room personnel should be familiar with the basic concepts and initial steps of these procedures. Failure to handle tissue appropriately may preclude the performance of needed diagnostic studies and ultimately delay or even prevent the establishment of a diagnosis. This chapter provides a basic introduction to the more common techniques employed in tissue fixation, staining, decalcification, and intraoperative consultation.

Fixation

Adequate fixation by an appropriate fixative is central to any histologic preparation. Tissue that is inadequately or inappropriately fixed will lead to difficulties in microtomy, staining and in performing ancillary tests. These problems may not be correctable at a later stage.

Unfortunately, there is no "all-purpose" fixative—no single fixative is good for all specimens. It is therefore essential that surgical pathology personnel be familiar with a variety of fixatives and their uses. Although the exact mechanism of action of many fixatives is unknown, fixatives can broadly be classified into four groups based on their mechanism of action. The aldehydes, such as formaldehyde and glutaraldehyde, act by cross-linking proteins, particularly lysine residues. Oxidizing agents, such as osmium tetroxide, potassium permanganate, and potassium dichromate, also probably cross-link proteins, although their precise mechanism of action is unknown. Acetic acid, methyl alcohol, and ethyl alcohol are all protein-denaturing agents. The fourth and final group of fixatives acts by the formation of insoluble metallic precipitates, and these include mercuric chloride and picric acid. The choice of the appropriate fixative is based on the type of tissue being fixed and on projected needs for ancillary tests such as special stains, immunohistochemistry, in situ hybridization, and electron microscopy. Table 2-1 lists some common fixatives, their basic uses, and their advantages and disadvantages.

Ten percent neutral buffered formalin (4% formaldehyde) is the standard fixative used in most laboratories. Formalin tends to remove water-soluble substances such as glycogen, and it is therefore generally not suitable for the fixation of tissues for electron microscopy. Ten percent neutral buffered formalin penetrates and fixes tissues at a rate of approximately 2 to 3 mm/24 h at room temperature.

Glutaraldehyde, a common fixative for electron microscopy, is one of the slowest penetrating fixatives. Tissue for electron microscopy should be cut into 1-mm cubes and immediately placed in refrigerated glutaraldehyde. Glutaraldehyde (4%) must be kept refrigerated before use.

Ethyl alcohol (70% to 100%) is seldom used as a primary fixative. It may be useful in fixing tissue for preserving glycogen and for some histochemical studies, but it has several disadvantages. Ethyl alcohol penetrates tissues very slowly, and because it denatures proteins by ab-

TABLE 2-1. Common fixatives.

Fixatives and their major components	Tissue	Special stains (+ = stain can be used with fixative) (− = stain should not be used with fixative)	Advantages (+) and disadvantages (−)
10% Neutral buffered formalin (4% Formaldehyde, 7.2 pH phosphate buffer, methanol)	All	+ Warthin-Starry (spirochetes) + Oil red O (fat) + Grimelius (neuroendocrine granules)	+ Routine fixative + Preservation, general staining + Immunohistochemistry + Molecular analyses + Long-term storage
2% Glutaraldehyde (50% Glutaraldehyde, 0.2 M cacodylate buffer)	All	− PAS (false positivity)	+ Electron microscopy + Preservation of collagen − Routine fixative − Slow penetration − Must be refrigerated
B5 (Mercuric chloride, sodium acetate, 37% formalin)	Lymph node Spleen Bone marrow		+ Cytoplasmic, nuclear staining − Routine fixative − Must be prepared fresh − Requires iodine treatment to remove mercury before routine staining − Timed exposure needed because overfixation causes hardening
Zenker's (Mercuric chloride, potassium dichromate, sodium sulfate, glacial acetic acid)	All	+ Sheehan (chromaffin) + Mallory's PTAH (collagen and muscle) + Viral inclusions (Negri bodies) + Feulgen (DNA) + Trichromes (collagen and muscle) + Verhoeff-van Gieson (elastic fibers)	+ Routine fixative + Preserves mitochondria − Must be washed overnight to remove excess chromate − Requires iodine treatment to remove mercury before routine staining − Must be prepared fresh − Molecular analyses − No metal instruments − Immunohistochemistry
Zenker's formol (Helly's fluid) (Mercuric chloride, potassium dichromate, sodium sulfate, 37% formaldehyde)	Bone marrow Spleen All blood-containing organs		+ Routine fixative + Preserves mitochondria + Preserves red blood cells − Must be washed overnight to remove chromate − Requires iodine treatment to remove mercury before routine staining − Molecular analyses − Immunohistochemistry
Bouin's (Picric acid, formalin, glacial acetic acid)	Testicular biopsies	+ Masson trichrome (collagen and muscle)	+ Routine fixative − Lyses red blood cells − Removes ferric iron − Dissolves some proteins − Molecular analyses − Immunohistochemistry − Carbohydrates

TABLE 2-1. *Continued.*

Fixatives and their major components	Tissue	Special stains (+ = stain can be used with fixative) (− = stain should not be used with fixative)	Advantages (+) and disadvantages (−)
Ethyl alcohol	All	+ Congo red (amyloid) + Von Kossa's (calcium) + Weigert's stain for fibrin + Mallory's stain for iron + Gomori's methenamine silver stain for urate crystals − Ziehl-Neelsen (AFB)	+ Enzyme histochemistry + Molecular analyses + Impression smears + Blood smears + Preserves glycogen + Preserves crystals: uric acid, sodium urate − Causes excessive hardening − Routine fixative − Dissolves lipids
Acetone 0–4°C	All	− Ziehl-Neelsen (AFB)	+ Enzyme histochemistry − Routine fixative − For best results, must be refrigerated − Dissolves lipids
Carnoy's (Glacial acetic acid, absolute ethanol, chloroform)	All	+ Methyl green pyronin (DNA and RNA) + Congo red (amyloid) + Giemsa (mast cells) − Ziehl-Neelsen (AFB)	+ Cytological fixative + Rapid penetration + Nuclear detail + Fixes RNA + Preserves glycogen − Dissolves cytoplasmic elements − Hemolyzes red blood cells

stracting water from the tissue, it can cause excessive hardening, tissue shrinkage, and cell distortion. Alcohol can also dissolve fats and should not be used when lipid studies or stains for myelin are being considered. Carnoy's is a fixative that combines ethanol, chloroform, and glacial acetic acid. It quickly fixes tissues and it is a good fixative for glycogen, plasma cells, and nucleic acids. Because of its quick action, some laboratories use Carnoy's to fix biopsies that require urgent processing.

The mercury-based fixatives (e.g., B5) provide excellent nuclear detail and are useful in evaluating lymphomas. Mercury-based fixatives precipitate proteins without firmly binding to them. These fixatives generally must be prepared fresh, and once fixed, the tissues require special processing in the histology laboratory (iodine treatment to remove the mercury). Overfixation with B5 can cause excessive hardening of the tissue.

Bouin's, a picric acid-based fixative, is the fixative of choice for testicular biopsies. Picric acid reacts with basic proteins and forms crystalline picrates with amino acids. Therefore, tissues fixed with picric acid-based fixatives retain little affinity for basic dyes, and the picric acid must be recovered from the tissue before staining. Picric acid penetrates tissues well and fixes them rapidly, but it also causes cells to shrink. Picric acid causes DNA methylation, hence, many polymerase chain reaction (PCR)-based molecular diagnostic tests cannot be performed on tissues fixed with picric acid.

The techniques of fixation are just as important as choosing the correct fixative. Appropriate fixation requires adequate tissue exposure and a duration sufficient to allow full penetration. To maximize the surface area of the specimen exposed to the fixative, lumina should be opened and solid tissues serially sectioned before fixation. The specimen can then be pinned to a wax block to maintain orientation and floated in a fixation tank. Paper towels can be placed in between sections to facilitate fixation. In general, the volume of fresh fixative should be at least 15 times the volume of the tissue. Most tissues are adequately fixed after 12 to 18 hours; however, adipose tissue, because of its hydrophobic nature, may require thinner sectioning and longer periods of fixation.

Special Stains

A variety of special stains are employed in the surgical pathology laboratory. Most of these are performed by specially trained laboratory personnel, and a detailed description of all of these stains is beyond the scope of this manual. The surgical pathologist and pathologist's assistant, however, should be able to perform a few basic stains—these include: the hematoxylin and eosin (H&E), oil red O (ORO), periodic acid-Schiff (PAS), Gram Weigert's (GW), Ziehl-Neelsen, and Papanicolaou (PAP) stains.

While the details of each stain vary from laboratory to laboratory, examples of "cookbook-style" instructions for the performance of each of these six stains on frozen tissue sections follow:

Stain: **Hematoxylin and Eosin (H&E)**

Approximate time: 3 minutes

Technique: 4 to 6 μm frozen section, touch prep, smear, crush prep

Any slides

Fixative: Absolute alcohol

Procedure:
1. Absolute alcohol, 60 seconds
2. Rinse in tap water (one change); dip until clear
3. Hematoxylin (Harris), 60 seconds
4. Rinse in tap water (three changes); dip until clear
5. Blue in Scott's water, 15 seconds
6. Rinse in tap water (two changes); dip until clear
7. Eosin-phloxine, 5 seconds
8. 50% Alcohol, five dips
9. 70% Alcohol, five dips
10. 95% Alcohol, five dips
11. Absolute alcohol, five dips (two changes)
12. Xylene (two changes); dip until clear
13. Mount and coverslip with resinous media

Results: Nuclei: blue to purple

Cytoplasm: pink to red

Stain: **Oil Red O (ORO)**

Approximate time: 10 minutes

Technique: 6 to 8 μm frozen section, touch prep, smear, crush prep

Poly-L-lysine or silanated slides

Fixative: 10% Neutral buffered formalin

Procedure:
1. 10% Neutral buffered formalin, 60 seconds
2. Wash in tap water and blot dry
3. Oil red O, 5 minutes
4. Wash in tap water
5. Hematoxylin (Harris), 60 seconds
6. Rinse in tap water (two changes)
7. Blue in Scott's water, 15 seconds
8. Rinse in tap water (two changes)
9. Mount and coverslip with *aqueous* media

Results: Fat: orange to bright red

Nuclei: blue

Cytoplasm: transparent

Stain: **Periodic Acid-Schiff (PAS)**

Approximate time: 35 minutes

Technique: 4 to 6 μm frozen section,

Poly-L-lysine or silanated slides

Fixative: Absolute alcohol

Procedure
1. Absolute alcohol, 60 seconds
2. Rinse in distilled water (one change)
3. 0.5% Periodic acid solution, 5 minutes
4. Rinse in distilled water (three changes)
5. Schiff reagent, 15 minutes
6. Wash in running tap water, 2 to 5 minutes or until pink color develops
7. Hematoxylin (Harris), 60 seconds
8. Wash in tap water, 2 minutes
9. 50% Alcohol, five dips
10. 70% Alcohol, five dips
11. 95% Alcohol, five dips (two changes)

12. Absolute alcohol, five dips (two changes)
13. Xylene (two changes); dip until clear
14. Mount and coverslip with resinous media

Results: Fungi: red to rose
Glycoproteins, mucopolysaccharides: red to rose
Nuclei: blue
Cytoplasm: light pink

Stain: **Gram Weigert's (GW)**
Approximate time: 10 minutes
Technique: 4 to 6 μm frozen section, touch prep, smear, crush prep
Poly-L-lysine or silanated slides
Fixative: Absolute alcohol
Procedure:
1. Absolute alcohol, 60 seconds
2. Eosin, 60 seconds
3. Rinse in tap water (one change)
4. Sterling's gentian violet, 60 seconds
5. Rinse in tap water (one change)
6. Gram's iodine, 2 minutes
7. Blot slides
8. Differentiate with aniline/ xylene mixture (two to three changes) until the black color is lost.
9. Xylene (two changes); dip until clear
10. Mount and coverslip with resinous media

Results: Gram-positive bacteria and *Pneumocystis carinii:* purple to blue
Nuclei: blue
Cytoplasm: light pink

Stain: **Modified Ziehl-Neelsen** (Acid Fast)
Approximate time: 60 minutes
Technique: 4 to 6 μm frozen section, Poly-L-lysine or silanated slides
Fixative: 10% Neutral Buffered Formalin (NBF)
Procedure:
1. Absolute alcohol, 60 seconds
2. Rinse in tap water

3. Carbol-fuchsin, 45 minutes
4. Wash in tap water
5. 1% Acid alcohol (one to two quick dips)
6. Wash in tap water
7. Methylene blue, 10 to 20 seconds
8. 50% Alcohol, five dips
9. 70% Alcohol, five dips
10. 90% Alcohol, five dips (two changes)
11. Absolute alcohol, five dips (two changes)
12. Xylene (two changes); dip until clear
13. Mount and cover slip with resinous media

Results: Acid-fast bacilli: bright red
Background: light blue

Stain: **Papanicolaou (PAP)**
Approximate time: 60 minutes
Technique: Touch prep, crush prep, smear, fine needle aspiration (FNA)
Poly-L-lysine or silanated slides
Fixative: 95% Alcohol
Procedure:
1. 95% Alcohol, 15 minutes
2. 75% Alcohol, five dips
3. 50% Alcohol, five dips
4. Distilled water, five dips
5. Hematoxylin, two to three minutes
6. Wash in tap water
7. 0.25% HCl, one to two quick dips
8. Wash in tap water
9. 30% Alcohol, five dips
10. 75% Alcohol, five dips
11. 95% Alcohol, five dips
12. Orange G, 2 minutes
13. 95% Alcohol, five dips (three changes)
14. Eosin-azure 50, 2 minutes
15. 95% Alcohol, five dips (two changes)
16. Xylene, five dips (three changes)
17. Mount and cover with resinous material

Results: Nuclei: blue
Cytoplasm: pink, gray, to green

Immunohistochemical Stains

Immunohistochemical studies employ an unlabeled antibody to a specific tissue antigen followed by treatment in one or more steps with an enzyme-labeled antibody. These studies are extremely versatile and can be used to detect an ever-expanding number of antigens. Depending on the specific antigens, they can be performed on fresh-frozen or formalin-fixed, paraffin-embedded tissues. The effectiveness of immunohistochemistry depends on the integrity, stability, and availability of the target antigen. Three steps can improve the results of your immunohistochemical staining. First, sample a viable and representative area of the process to be studied. Immunohistochemical stains of necrotic material are practically worthless. Second, choose the appropriate method of stabilizing the tissue. While formalin is generally a good fixative for most immunohistochemical stains, some stains work best in other fixatives, and other stains work only on fresh-frozen tissue. Finally, do not overfix the tissue. Overfixation may result in the loss of antigenicity.

Decalcification

A wide variety of calcified specimens are received in the surgical pathology laboratory. While some of these should be cut with specialized, expensive equipment, the vast majority of calcified specimens can be handled by a routine histology laboratory if they are appropriately decalcified. Decalcification is the process whereby calcium salts are removed from bone and other calcified tissues. Three general methods are employed to decalcify tissues. These include acid hydrolysis, organic chelation, and electrolysis (see Table 2-2). The important points to remember about decalcifying specimens follow:

1. The tissue must be fixed before decalcification. In most cases, fixing a specimen for at least 24 hours in 10% neutral buffered formalin is adequate. If you use a different fixative, make sure that the fixative employed is compatible with the method of decalcification chosen.

2. Decalcification should be carried out at room temperature and with constant magnetic stirring. While heat accelerates decalcification, it also induces numerous artifacts and thus should be avoided.

3. Do not decalcify longer than necessary, as excessive decalcification will introduce artifacts. To avoid overdecalcification, delicate tissues should be examined every hour, and larger tissues as established by laboratory protocol.

4. Residual acid will destroy nuclear detail. Therefore, acid decalcification solutions must be removed from bone specimens before they are processed by washing them in water for at least 24 hours.

5. The volume of the decalcification solution should be 10 to 15 times that of the tissue being decalcified. These solutions should also be changed on a regular basis.

Intraoperative Consultation

Important decisions in the operating room are frequently based on intraoperative consultation with a pathologist. These intraoperative consultations often require the rapid microscopic examination of fresh tissue. This examination can be accomplished either by the preparation of cytologic slides or by the preparation of histologic slides using the frozen section technique.

Cytologic slides can be prepared from fresh specimens by one of three methods. Impression smears are produced by touching a microscopic slide to the cut face of the tissue. This procedure is also known as a touch preparation. The slide can be air dried or immediately fixed in alcohol for subsequent staining. The crush preparation is performed by taking a small (1-mm cube) piece of tissue and crushing it between two glass slides. The crush preparation can be fixed or air dried, then stained. Extremely hard tissues can be *scraped* with a sharp blade and the scrapings drawn across another slide in much the same way that a blood smear is prepared. Each of these techniques can be used on different tissues with varying degrees of success in terms of preparation artifacts and quantity of cells obtained. For example, crush preparations work best on very soft tissues, while scrapings are needed on very firm tissues.

TABLE 2-2. Acid decalcification methods.

Decalcification method	Tissue	Comment	Advantages (+) and disadvantages (−)
Acid hydrolysis, 3% HCl	Routine decalcification of cortical bone, large thick bone, ossified cancellous bone	Compatible with most routine and special staining methods May interfere with immunoperoxidase and other special studies Method of choice for large specimens	± Immunohistochemistry − Swells cells − Overdecalcification results in extreme eosinophilia
Acid hydrolysis, 5% HNO₃	Routine decalcification of cortical bone, large thick bone, ossified cancellous bone	Compatible with most routine and special staining methods, but yields substandard results	− Damages nuclear detail − Immunohistochemistry − Swells cells
Acid hydrolysis, 5% formic acid	Light decalcification of delicate tissue, bone marrow, bones of inner ear	Compatible with most routine and special staining methods Method of choice for small specimens	+ Immunohistochemistry + Good preservation of nuclear detail

The frozen section is another procedure frequently used in intraoperative consultations. The details of preparing a frozen section vary greatly from one laboratory to another; however, one should become familiar with a few general concepts.

The first step is to select and prepare a piece of the specimen to freeze. Select a section that demonstrates the interface of the lesion with normal tissue, and try to avoid fatty or calcified tissues. The section should not be greater than 2 × 2 cm, and wet tissue should be gently blotted dry to avoid the formation of ice crystals. Very small pieces are easily lost in opaque embedding medium, so they should be stained with a drop of eosin or India ink before sectioning.

The second step is to freeze the tissue. Tissues are usually frozen on a tissue chuck in freezing medium by immersion in liquid nitrogen. This technique will lead to the formation of ice crystals, which can distort the histology. Some laboratories therefore prefer to use either refrigerated units with isopentane or cryostats equipped with specialized heat extractors.

Once the specimen is frozen, it is ready for sectioning. A variety of sectioning artifacts can be reduced with a few simple tricks. For example, sections that have been overly frozen will crumble when sectioned. In these cases, simply warm up the block by pressing a gloved thumb firmly onto its surface. (Be careful not to cut your finger on the cryostat blade.) Inadequate freezing, on the other hand, will cause the sections to stick and bind. In these cases, the specimen can be frozen to the appropriate temperature using a cooling spray, such as Histofreeze. Lines and knife marks can be avoided by using a clean and extremely sharp blade. Finally, loosely set screws can contribute to vibration artifacts, so if the sections look like corduroy pants, tighten all of the screws holding the block.

Once the section has been cut, it should be placed on a glass slide, fixed, and stained. A variety of stains are employed in different laboratories (see earlier for the H&E technique), but whichever stains are used, remember to take your time and follow the staining protocol. Too frequently, staining procedures are rushed, and the slides to be stained barely touch the staining solution. The resultant slides can be impossible to interpret or, ironically, may take longer to interpret than a slide stained correctly. Also, when one rushes, one often transfers solutions from one Coplin jar to the next. As a result, solutions are contaminated, and the quality of subsequent frozen sections is diminished. This problem can be reduced simply to touching the edge of the slide to the edge of the jar before transferring the slide to a new solution. Another problem encountered during staining is that tissue can fall off of the slide. If this happens, try using silanated or other specially treated slides. The ultimate goal in preparation of a frozen section is to render a timely and accurate intraoperative diagnosis. Remember to save the piece of tissue that was frozen so that it can serve as a frozen section control for diagnostic and quality control purposes.

3 Photography

Norman J. Barker, M.S., R.B.P.

Quality gross specimen photographs are an essential part of surgical pathology. Aesthetically pleasing 35-mm color slides and black-and-white prints are used not only to document the diagnosis but also for conferences, presentations, teaching, and publications. Unfortunately, photographs are often not taken, or if they are taken, they are not useful because of underexposure, overexposure, inappropriate lighting, poor selection of background, or blood-stained or -smeared backgrounds. Fortunately, with care and a standardized system, you can produce consistent high-quality photographs. This chapter first describes how to set up a standard photographic system and then describes how to photograph specimens and troubleshoot a variety of problems.

Setting Up a Photographic System

Photographic Stand

A variety of camera stands are on the market. Pick one with a sturdy column. Sturdy columns eliminate camera vibration, which causes photographs to be out of focus. Probably the most versatile and easy to use system on the market is the Polaroid MP4, which consists of a heavy-duty stand, a 4 × 5-inch camera, and permanently mounted but adjustable lighting (Fig. 3-A). It also has an adapter for a 35-mm camera. With this system, Polaroid 4 × 5-inch black-and-white negative film can be used to produce an instant print and negative. The print serves as an instant record, documenting the size and condition of the specimen, and notes can be made directly on the print, providing a visual correlate of the gross description. The negative can be filed and prints for publication made from it at a future date.

Lens Selection

Most major camera manufacturers offer a choice of two types of macro lenses. The 60-mm macro lens is sufficient for 95% of routine work in the surgical pathology laboratory. The 105-mm macro lens allows for more working distance between the specimen and the front of the lens. This feature is helpful when doing close-up work. Both of these macro lenses are extremely useful because they can focus down to a point where the image on the negative is the same size as the specimen, and they will cover specimens ranging in size from a large colon down to small polyps. One of the scales that is not present on most ordinary lenses, but that is printed on macro lenses, is the reproduction ratio. You should be familiar with this scale because, as discussed later, it can be used to determine the appropriate exposure for a specimen (Fig. 3-B).

Background Selection

Before lighting the subject, background selection must be considered. The correct background will enhance and highlight the subject to be photographed. A background table can be easily made or commercially purchased. The latter is a good choice but is only good for medium to small specimens. The Aristo Box DA-17 (Fig. 3-C) has a cool rectangular, fluorescent light inside. The box gives a flat shadowless illu-

Fig. 3-A. The Polaroid MP4 system.

Film T-64 60-mm macro lens		
F-Stop	Time (s)	Reproduction Ratio
22 ½	¼	1 : 10
22	¼	1 : 7
16 ½	¼	1 : 3
16	¼	1 : 1

Fig. 3-B. Example of a gross stand exposure chart. Create a chart such as this one to calculate the f-stop when doing close-up work. The reproduction ratio value is printed on most lenses.

Fig. 3-C. Aristo DA-17 light box.

Fig. 3-D. Custom background box.

Fig. 3-E. Standard flat copy lighting.

Fig. 3-F. Side lighting—texture.

Fig. 3-G. Fiber-optic lighting—cavity.

mination or, if turned upside down, a black background.

A more versatile system (Fig. 3-D) can be custom made to fit space requirements. A custom background box should have even fluorescent lighting below a glass surface on which specimens can be placed. Immediately on top of the fluorescent lights is a place for opal glass or Plexiglas, which diffuses the light for an even background. Colored gels can then be placed on top of the Plexiglas for a variety of background selections. There is then a space of about 6 to 8 inches between the background and the specimen glass. This system eliminates shadows on the background.

If colored gels are used for backgrounds, great care must be taken. An ill-chosen background color can affect the color of the specimen in the photograph. For many specimens, red, yellow, and green are colors to avoid. Shooting an actual test photograph is the only way to tell for sure. One very simple type of background is a piece of black velvet available in fabric shops. This material will absorb all light that falls on it, yielding a pure black background. Therefore no shadows from the specimen will be seen. A solid black background also has the advantage of hiding liquids that have seeped out from a specimen. This makes a cleaner presentation in the final photograph.

Lighting

Important features of a specimen may be hidden when the lighting is too dim or obscured when the lighting is too bright. Appropriate lighting, on the other hand, will actually enhance the photographic demonstration of these findings. One of the many advantages of the Polaroid MP4 stand is the fact that the lights may be easily moved to highlight the features of a particular specimen. Lights placed in the standard 45° position (standard copy lighting) provide an even, flat illumination for the majority of specimens (Fig. 3-E).

The standard 45° positioning of the light source may not be optimal for every specimen. For example, when three-dimensional information is most important, the lights should be positioned at a lower angle (Fig. 3-F). This will provide shadows that will help suggest a relief or delineate form from its background. This po-

sitioning of the light source can help show texture as well. Another technique is to unplug the lights on one side, so that a stronger contrast can be seen. The main thing to keep in mind is that lighting should not obscure information.

A good addition to a lighting system is a fiber-optic light source (Fig. 3-G). Manipulable fiber optic wands provide an excellent source of illumination when close-ups are required. They are particularly useful in illuminating cavities and crevices. When used in combination with other light sources, fiber-optic lights are also effective in "filling in" otherwise darkened areas. Keep in mind that when lighting changes are made, some changes in exposure may also be necessary.

Thirty-Five–Millimeter Slides

Not only can 35-mm slides be used for projection at conferences, they can be used for publication as well. The slides also can be scanned into a computer, and letters, numbers, or arrows may be added. Other slides can be scanned and combined together, such as a gross and microscopic view on one slide. A 35-mm slide may be converted to a black-and-white print for publication.

Color slides are best obtained with a 35-mm single-lens-reflex camera with through-the-lens light metering. The best results are achieved with fine-grain films. A film should be selected for accurate color rendition, and it should match the Kelvin temperature of the lights used. Most gross specimen photography is done with tungsten halogen lamps (3200 K) as opposed to an electronic flash (5500 K). Unlike the transient illumination of the electronic flash, tungsten lamps provide constant illumination so that the lighting can be critically evaluated before the photograph is taken. Kodak Ektachrome tungsten EPY-64 is a good choice of film. This film is balanced for tungsten lamps, it has a high resolution, tends to match the true specimen colors, and is a user-processed film. (User-processed film can be processed at most hospital in-house photographic departments, usually on a same-day basis.) Films such as Kodachrome, on the other hand, tend to enhance red and yellow colors and must be sent to outside labs for processing.

Standardized Exposure Determination

The amount of light that reaches the film can be controlled in two ways. One is to change the aperture. The *aperture* refers to the diameter of the lens diaphragm, and this can be adjusted by changing the f-stop. Each f-stop setting changes the amount of light passing through the lens by a factor of 2. The smaller the f-stop number, the larger the aperture and the more open the lens. For example, an f-stop of 2 will let more light into the camera than an f-stop of 22. The aperture also controls the *depth of field*, which refers to the zone of sharpness in front of and behind the point of focus. With large apertures (smaller f-stop numbers), everything outside the plane of focus abruptly becomes blurred. At very small apertures (such as an f-stop of 22), objects remain in focus over a greater depth of field. Therefore, optimal clarity is best achieved using a smaller aperture (higher f-stop).

The amount of light hitting the film is also controlled by the shutter speed. The *shutter speed* refers to the length of time that the lens is open. Each shutter speed, like the f-stop, doubles or halves the exposure at the next setting. Standard speeds on modern shutters are 1, ½, ¼, ⅛, 1/15, 1/30, 1/60, 1/125 second, etc. Keep in mind that both the aperture and shutter control the amount of light falling on the film

You need to identify the best f-stops and shutter speeds for your particular system by running a series of exposure tests for each different specimen magnification. To do this, you need a light meter. An incident light meter works best because it measures the light falling on the specimen. The reflected light meters that are found in most cameras can be "fooled" and give incorrect readings because of the light coming from the background. For example, reflected light meters may read too much of the background and not enough of the specimen when a lightly colored specimen on a black background is being photographed. Once the exposure is approximated with the hand-held incident light meter, a series of test exposures should be made at different magnifications (reproduction ratios). Most manufactured lenses have reproduction ratios listed on the lens barrel for each magnification. In making this test run, choose a standard exposure such as ¼ second, and then vary the aperture of the camera by one half of an f-stop at each magnification. This exposure time will enable you to use small apertures, which result in a better depth of field and translate into better specimen focus. The best aperture then can be determined for a specific image magnification, and a chart can be made listing the correct aperture that matches each magnification (Fig. 3-B). While this system is easy to use, it may be necessary to modify the exposure for very dark blood-red specimens or very light white specimens.

Scale

While many find scales and labels unnecessary distracters in an otherwise aesthetic photograph, at least one of the specimen photographs should include a scale along with the specimen identification number. A scale helps the viewer orient the specimen and provides a benchmark for the perception of size, while specimen labeling ensures that the photographs will not be lost or misidentified later. Commercially prepared plastic rulers are available that can be made into various sizes to accommodate different specimens. Small adhesive labels with the specimen identification number can be attached directly to the ruler. When placing the scale in a photograph, be sure to place it in the anatomical inferior position. The scale should be positioned at the level of the specimen so that it is in plane of focus.

Some Pointers on Photographing Specimens

General Principles

A few simple steps will improve the aesthetic quality of your photographs. First, photograph the cut surface of the specimen. A photograph of the external surface of a specimen is seldom informative. Section the specimen using a fluid sweeping motion to create a cut surface that is smooth and unruffled. Take the photograph before gouging out tissue for frozen section evaluation or tumor collection; or if these studies are urgently needed, take the tissue from an area that will not be shown in the photograph. Gently rinse blood and fluid from the surface of the specimen, and then blot the surface of the specimen dry so that fluid does not seep across the field of view.

Second, decide whether the pathology is best demonstrated in the specimen before or after it is fixed. Color is best seen when the specimen is photographed fresh, while fine structural details are sometimes better appreciated in fixed specimens, which reflect less light.

Third, position the specimen so that (1) the area of interest is centered in the field of view; (2) its long axis is oriented along the long axis of the frame; and (3) the specimen fills at least 75% of the frame. For bivalved specimens, there is no need to photograph both halves of the specimen. Instead, fill the frame with a closer view of just one of the two halves. To point out a focal area of interest, use a clean and unassuming probe or pointer (not a finger).

Fourth, make sure the background is clean and free of distracters. Remember that your work is not over once the photograph is taken. Remove the specimen, and clean the background so that it is ready for the next user.

Dark Specimens

Many fresh specimens and bloody specimens tend to produce dark images on film. As a general rule, you can compensate by opening the lens by one f-stop (decrease the f-stop number). This will lighten the specimen in the final photograph.

Light Specimens

Photographs of fixed specimens can sometimes be bleached white with little or no color information. Try taking one photograph at the normal exposure. Then take several more photographs while increasing the f-stop number in half increments (e.g., f-stop 16, 16½, 22, etc.) This intentional closing of the lens and consequent underexposure should provide more detail in the very light areas.

Large Specimens

Large specimens generally require at least two sets of photographs—one of the entire specimen and the other a close-up of the area of interest.

The close-up photograph will demonstrate the finer details of a lesion, while the overall view will show the relationship of the lesion to the rest of the specimen.

Small Specimens

Most normal lenses will not focus when moved very close (i.e., within 2 feet) to the specimen. A special macro lens is needed for very small specimens or for close-up photographs to show fine detail. The 105-mm macro lens is especially suitable for these purposes. It can focus to a point where the image on the negative is the same size as the specimen, while maintaining a comfortable working distance between the front of the lens and the specimen. Remember that focus is critical in close-up work. Even small specimens can have depth, so avoid focusing only on the top of the specimen by focusing on a point about one third of the way down from the top of the specimen. Also, use a small camera aperture (an f-stop of 22) for increased depth of field.

Oddly Shaped Specimens

Oddly shaped specimens are a nuisance to photograph when they cannot be maintained in the correct position. A simple solution is modeling clay, which can be used to prop up the specimen. Mold the clay into shape, and use it as a base to hold the specimen. Before taking the picture, be sure to look through the viewfinder to make sure that the clay will not show up in the final photograph. Small fish hooks with nylon cord and an attached weight can be used to hold areas open. For example, this technique can be useful when photographing the interior of heart valves.

Cavities

Under standard lighting conditions, the walls of a cavity cast shadows that obscure the base of the cavity. To circumvent this problem, place the lights as high as possible, so that they illuminate the depths of the cavity. This type of vertical illumination will help reduce shadows as well as light the entire cavity. A separate fiber-optic light source can also be of great help.

Make sure that you are focused on the area of interest because depth of field can be a problem.

Three-Dimensional Structures

Side lighting is the best lighting to demonstrate surface detail or to show the three-dimensional quality of a tumor. The lower the angle of the light, the more surface relief will be seen. Shadows give the form shape, depth, and contrast. Be careful not to set the lights too low, as this can create harsh shadows that obscure detail.

Troubleshooting

Reflection

If you are using a piece of glass to support the specimen, watch out for reflections. A valuable photograph can be ruined when overhead (ceiling) lights, the photographer's hand, or the photographer's face is seen reflected in the background. Always use a cable release (the extender cable that allows the photographer to trigger the shutter from a distance), not only to keep the camera still, but also to avoid reflections in the glass. Fixed specimens reflect much less light than fresh specimens. If the specimen is fresh, reflected light can be reduced by drying the surface of the specimen with a paper towel. Before tripping the shutter, look through the viewfinder and study the field. Make sure that the lighting and arrangement best demonstrate the pathology of interest.

Exposure

Once an exposure test has been made and an exposure chart posted, the camera should consistently produce uniform high-quality exposures. A photograph that is too light is likely due to overexposure. The simple solution is to close the aperture. (For example, an f-stop setting of 11 can be changed to a setting of 16 or 22.) If the photograph is too dark, simply open the aperture so that the film receives more light. With a little practice and a standard system, you should be well on the way to top-quality specimen photographs.

Maintenance of the Photography System

Not surprisingly, a system designed for use by many users is particularly susceptible to abuse and neglect. Proper maintenance of a photography system is a daily task that is less likely to be neglected if assigned to one person. This person should be responsible for: maintaining clean lenses and viewfinders as well as a fresh supply of film; checking that the cameras are loaded with film; and checking that the film is delivered for processing in a timely fashion. There is nothing worse than spending valuable time in photographing an important specimen and afterward finding out that there was no film in the camera!

Things to Remember when Photographing a Specimen

- Always make sure the background is clean. A spray bottle and towels should be part of the photography setup.
- Orient the specimen. Mark the specimen with a proper identification tag, and include a scale in the plane of focus.
- Always use a cable release to eliminate unwanted camera vibration and reflection.
- Double-check the focus and exposure settings.
- Verify that the lighting shows what you want. Take great care to avoid shadows that obscure features of particular interest.

Commercial Products/ Equipment Vendors

1. Aristo DA-17 Light Box: Aristo Grids Lamp Products, 65 Harbor Rd., P.O. Box 769, Port Washington, NY 11050.
2. Polaroid MP4 Camera: Polaroid Corp., 575 Technology Square, Cambridge, MA 02139.
3. Copy stands and view boxes: Kinex, 34 Elton Street, Rochester, NY 14607.
4. 150-mm Rulers (Cat. No. 09-016): Fisher Scientific Co., 711 Forbes Ave., Pittsburgh, PA 25219.

II The Head and Neck

4 Larynx

The Anatomy

The patterns of spread of carcinomas of the larynx depend on their site of origin and on well-defined anatomic barriers. A detailed understanding of laryngeal anatomy is therefore an essential part of the dissection of any laryngeal specimen. Take time to look over the figures and refresh your memory of laryngeal anatomy.

The most important thing to remember about laryngal anatomy is that the larynx is composed of three anatomic regions: the supraglottis, the glottis, and the subglottis. The supraglottis is the portion of the larynx superior to the ventricles. It is composed of the epiglottis, the arytenoids, the aryepiglottic folds, and the false cords. The glottis is composed of the true vocal cords and their anterior and posterior attachments, the anterior and posterior commissures. The subglottis begins 1 cm below the free edge of the vocal cords and extends inferiorly to the trachea. These three anatomic regions should be kept in mind throughout your description and dissection of the larynx.

The important mucosal landmarks to identify in the larynx are illustrated and include the mucosa overlying the base of the tongue, the epiglottis, the aryepiglottic folds, the pyriform sinuses, the false vocal cords, the ventricles, and the true vocal cords. These mucosal surfaces cover the cartilaginous framework of the larynx. This framework includes the cartilage of the epiglottis, the thyroid cartilage, and the cricoid cartilage. The epiglottis is attached to the thyroid cartilage by the thyroepiglottic ligament. The shield-shaped thyroid cartilage forms the anterior and lateral walls of the larynx. The cricoid cartilage is shaped like a signet ring, and it forms the posterior wall of the larynx. Situated in the back of the larynx are the two arytenoid cartilages. These are pyramidal in shape and rest along the upper border of the cricoid cartilage. Although the hyoid bone is not technically part of the larynx, it is often included in laryngectomy specimens.

Three additional anatomic landmarks need to be defined because cancers that invade these landmarks frequently escape from the larynx. The *pre-epiglottic space* is the triangular space anterior to the base of the epiglottis. The pre-epiglottic space is filled with fatty connective tissue, and it is bounded posteriorly by the epiglottis, inferiorly by the thyroepiglottic ligament, anteriorly by the thyrohyoid membrane, and superiorly by the hyoepiglottic ligament. The *paraglottic space* is a less well-defined area composed of loose connective tissue, which lies between the thyroid cartilage and two membranes that form the structural base for the vocal folds, the conus elasticus and quadrangular membrane. The *anterior commissure* is the anterior dense ligamentous attachment of the true vocal cords to the thyroid cartilage. The thyroid cartilage lacks an internal perichondrium; therefore, carcinomas may invade the thyroid cartilage at the level of the anterior commissure. Carcinomas may also escape the larynx inferiorly via the cricothyroid membrane.

Finally, although the pyriform sinuses are technically part of the hypopharynx, one should be aware of them because they are frequently resected with the larynx. The pyriform sinuses are small pouches that extend inferiorly from the intersection of the aryepiglottic folds, glossoepiglottic folds, and pharyngeal wall.

Total Laryngectomy

The easiest way to orient a total laryngectomy specimen is to identify the epiglottis. The epiglottis is present anteriorly at the most superior aspect of the larynx, and the flap of the epiglottis closes posteriorly. If the epiglottis is not present, then the thyroid cartilage can be used to orient the specimen. The superior horns of the thyroid cartilage are located superiorly and project posteriorly, while the V-shaped apex of the thyroid cartilage points anteriorly.

After the specimen has been oriented, ink the soft tissue and mucosal margins. The mucosal margins essentially form two rings. The inferior ring is formed by the trachea, and the superior ring is formed by the circular opening of the larynx into the pharynx. After the margins have been inked, cut through the posterior wall of the larynx in the midline using a pair of scissors. This posterior midline approach will fully expose the mucosal surfaces of the larynx without disrupting the anatomic structures located along its anterior and internal walls. The larynx can then be cracked open posteriorly by expanding the posterior opening with your thumbs. The easiest and safest way to do this is to push hard on the superior horns of the thyroid cartilage. The posterior aspect of the larynx can then be kept open using a small wooden stick. The opened larynx should be photographed and the specimen fixed overnight in formalin.

Once the specimen is fixed, the mucosal margins can be sampled. Sampling the inferior mucosal margin is a relatively simple step. If this margin is not closely approached by tumor, it can be taken as a single shave section of the tracheal stump. If the tumor is close to the inferior margin, take perpendicular sections. Sampling the superior mucosal margin, on the other hand, is much more labor intensive. This mucosal margin spans a number of important laryngeal structures, and great care must be taken to both sample the margin thoroughly and to designate each sampled margin as precisely as possible. As illustrated, the superior mucosal margin is formed (1) anteriorly by the mucosa of the base of the tongue, (2) laterally by the pyriform sinuses or lateral hypopharyngeal walls, and (3) posteriorly by the posterior cricoid mucosa, which is the anterior hypopharyngeal

wall. Perpendicular sections of each of these three mucosal margins should be taken. Next, take the soft tissue margins. These can be taken as perpendicular sections from the anterior surface of the specimen and from any other areas where the soft tissues appear infiltrated by tumor.

Once all the margins are taken, turn your attention to the tumor. Keeping the three anatomic regions of the larynx (the supraglottis, glottis, and subglottis) in mind, carefully document the side, size, and exact location of any tumors. Also note whether the tumor is endophytic or exophytic. Submit sections of each identified tumor for histology to show its maximal depth of invasion as well as its relationship to grossly uninvolved mucosa. Next, carefully examine, document, and sample for histology the mucosa of the pyriform sinuses, the epiglottis, the aryepiglottic folds, the false cords, the ventricles, the true vocal cords, the anterior commissure, and the subglottis. In general, longitudinal sections are most informative. As illustrated, a single longitudinal section can be taken to include the false cord, the ventricle, and the true cord. Carefully examine and sample for histology the thyroid cartilage (especially deep to the tumor), the cricoid cartilage, and the hyoid bone. These sections may have to be submitted for decalcification. If a tracheostomy site is present, it should be noted, and several sections of it should be submitted for histologic examination. Finally, remember the three additional anatomic landmarks discussed earlier. The pre-epiglottic space can be sampled by taking a midline section from the base of the epiglottis superiorly and anteriorly toward the hyoid bone. As illustrated, the paraglottic space is usually included in the histologic section of the true and false cords. Finally, a section of the anterior commissure should be submitted in cancers that involve the vocal cords.

If any organs were removed along with the larynx, then their presence should be documented. Be especially diligent in your search for the thyroid gland. Often, only a portion of the gland is removed with the larynx, and it may be embedded within the anterior soft tissues and strap muscles. If the thyroid gland is present, examine it as described in the thyroid section (Chapter 32) and remember to look for parathyroid glands. If a radical neck dissection is attached, it can be removed and examined sepa-

Pyriform
sinus

Epiglottis

Hyoid bone

Aryepiglottic
fold

Superior horn
of the thyroid
cartilage

Ink the exposed soft tissues,
and open the posterior surface
of the larynx.

Epiglottis

Section of
pre-epiglottic
space

Base of tongue

Hyoid
bone

Supraglottis

False cord

Ventricle

Glottis

True cord

Thyroid cartilage

Subglottis

Cricoid
cartilage

Although this is a plane of section you will not see,
we find this diagram helpful, because it demonstrates
the anatomy and the location of the pre-epiglottic space.

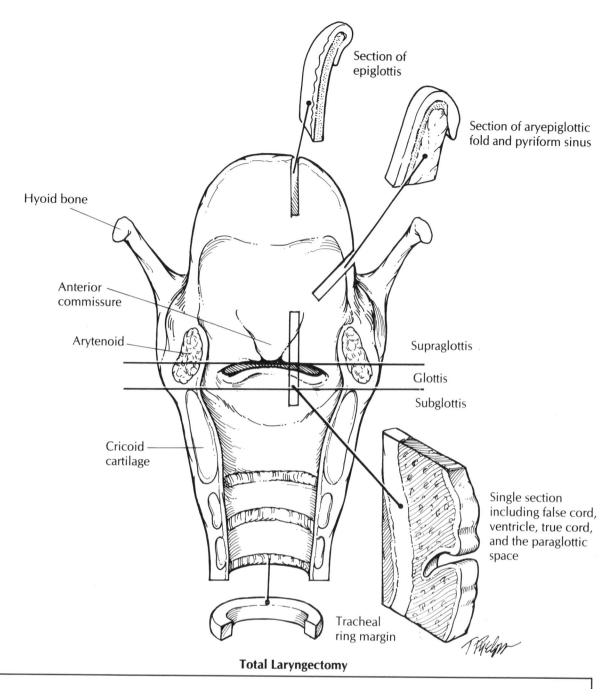

Section of epiglottis

Section of aryepiglottic fold and pyriform sinus

Hyoid bone

Anterior commissure

Arytenoid

Supraglottis

Glottis

Subglottis

Cricoid cartilage

Single section including false cord, ventricle, true cord, and the paraglottic space

Tracheal ring margin

Total Laryngectomy

1. Orient the specimen. The epiglottis is present anteriorly at the most superior aspect of the larynx, and the flap of the epiglottis closes posteriorly.

2. Ink the margins, and then cut through the posterior wall of the larynx in the midline. Open the larynx by pushing hard on the superior horns of the thyroid cartilage.

3. Submit sections of the inferior (tracheal) and superior (base of tongue, pyriform sinus or lateral hypopharyngeal wall, and posterior cricoid) mucosal margins and anterior and posterior soft tissue margins.

4. Describe and submit sections of the tumor, keeping the three anatomic regions of the larynx in mind: the supraglottis, the glottis, and the subglottis.

5. Submit a section from both sides to include the false cords, the ventricles, and the true cords. Submit sections of the pyriform sinuses, the epiglottis, the aryepiglottic folds, the anterior commissure, the subglottis, the thyroid cartilage, the cricoid cartilage, and the hyoid bone. Submit sections of the pre-epiglottic space, the paraglottic space, and the anterior commissure.

rately as described in the section on radical neck dissections (Chapter 7).

Subtotal Laryngectomies

Portions of the larynx can also be resected. For example, a *hemilaryngectomy* is a voice-preserving procedure in which either the left or right thyroid cartilage, true vocal cord, false cord, and ventricle are removed in continuity. A *supraglottic laryngectomy* is a procedure performed for tumors of the supraglottic larynx in which the supraglottis is removed with a horizontal incision through the ventricles. The approach to these subtotal laryngectomy specimens should follow that for total laryngectomies. In addition, the new margins created by the procedure need to be sampled.

Important Issues to Address in Your Surgical Pathology Report on the Larynx*

General

- What procedure was performed, and what structures/organs are present?
- What is the exact location of the tumor?
- What are the tumor's size, grade, type, and growth pattern (exophytic or endophytic)?
- Is there perineural and/or vascular invasion?
- Are any soft tissue or mucosal margins involved?

---

*Modified from Kirchner JA, Carter D. The larynx. In: Sternberg SS, ed. *Diagnostic Surgical Pathology*, 2nd ed. New York: Raven Press; 1994:907–908.

Supraglottic Cancers

- If the hyoid bone is attached, is the tumor above or below the level of the hyoid?
- Does the tumor involve the false cord, the epiglottis, the aryepiglottic folds, and/or the arytenoids?
- Does the inferior edge of the tumor involve the anterior commissure and/or the roof of the ventricle?
- If the aryepiglottic fold is involved, how far down the pyriform sinus does the tumor extend?
- How far does the cancer extend superiorly toward the base of the tongue?
- Does the cancer involve the pre-epiglottic space?
- Does the tumor invade the cartilaginous framework?

Glottic Cancers

- Does the tumor involve one vocal cord or both, and what is the length of the cord involvement?
- Is the anterior commissure involved? If so, does the tumor extend anteriorly into the thyroid cartilage?
- How far inferiorly below the free edge of the true vocal cords does the tumor extend (in millimeters)?
- Does the tumor extend superiorly into the ventricle, false cord, or base of the epiglottis?
- Does the cancer involve the paraglottic space?

Subglottic Cancers

- What is the superior extent of the tumor? Does it involve the true vocal cord?
- What is the inferior extent of the tumor? How close is the tumor to the inferior margin?
- What is the maximal depth of invasion? Does the carcinoma penetrate the conus elasticus and extend into the paraglottic space?

5 Salivary Glands

The gross appearance of some salivary gland neoplasms is so characteristic that one can come close to establishing the diagnosis on the gross findings alone. Yet, all too often, salivary glands are simply inked, bread-loafed, and thrown into tissue cassettes. Take time to describe the appearance of any lesions encountered.

Examine the external surface of the specimen after it has been weighed and measured. Carefully look for and tag with safety pins any large nerves that may have been resected with the gland. It is important to sample these nerves for histology, but they will not be identifiable after the specimen has been inked. Next, ink the specimen, and section the gland at 2- to 3-mm intervals. Measure the size of any tumors encountered, and describe their gross appearance. Are they well demarcated and encapsulated or poorly demarcated and infiltrative? Is the tumor solid or cystic? Are areas of cartilaginous differentiation appreciable grossly? How close is the tumor to the margins? Next, submit the entire tumor for histologic examination. Do not just scoop out the center of the tumor; instead, carefully submit sections showing the relationship of the tumor to the inked soft tissue margin, of the tumor to the adjacent uninvolved gland, and as noted, of the tumor to any grossly identifiable nerves. Once the tumor has been described and submitted for histology, the rest of the gland can be examined and described. Are any calculi present, and are the ducts of the salivary gland dilated? Submit a representative section of grossly uninvolved salivary gland. Finally, the soft tissue around the gland should be examined, and a representative section of each identified lymph node should be submitted.

Important Issues to Address in Your Surgical Pathology Report on Salivary Glands

- What procedure was performed, and what structures/organs are present?
- Is a neoplasm present?
- What are the type, size, and degree of differentiation of the tumor?
- Does the tumor infiltrate small or large nerves?
- Does the tumor involve any of the margins?
- If lymph nodes are present, how many are present, and how many are involved by tumor?
- Does the non-neoplastic portion of the salivary gland show any pathology?

6 Complex Specimens

Treat nature in terms of the cylinder, the sphere, and the cone, all in perspective.
Cézanne

While we have attempted to illustrate the dissection of the majority of the standard head and neck specimens received in the surgical pathology laboratory, you will occasionally be faced with a complex specimen that we have not illustrated. Without a game plan, these specimens can be overwhelming.

Our approach is a simple one based on four steps. First, identify the various components of the specimen (epithelium, bone, soft tissue, etc.). Second, think of each component as a geometric shape. Third, approach each component separately. Fourth, look for the relationships between any lesions and each component. This approach is illustrated below with the dissection of a portion of the tongue and mandible (partial glossectomy with partial mandibulectomy) resected for cancer.

Step 1.
Identify the Various Components of the Specimen

In this case, the components include the soft tissue and muscle of the tongue, the epithelium of the oral cavity, and the bone of the mandible. This step helps ensure that important components of the specimen are not left out of the dissection, gross description, and tissue sampled for histology.

Step 2.
Think of Each Component as a Geometric Shape

For example, as illustrated for the partial glossectomy with partial mandibulectomy specimen, the muscle of the tongue can be thought of as a cube, the bone of the mandible as a cylinder, and the epithelium as a flat two-dimensional square sheet.

Step 3.
Approach Each Component Separately

The goal here is to take sections that will demonstrate each margin. The margins are easily remembered using the geometric shapes visualized for each component. For example, the muscle is thought of as a cube. You should therefore take perpendicular margins from each face of the cube. As illustrated, these include the anterior, posterior, medial, lateral, and inferior surfaces. The sixth surface, the superior surface, is covered by the epithelium, so this is not a margin. Similarly, the epithelium is thought of as a square sheet. Take perpendicular margins from the posterior, anterior, medial, and lateral edges of this square. Finally, the bone is thought of as a cylinder. Shave sections of the two ends of the

Bone—think of it as a cylinder.

Epithelium—treat it as a square sheet.

The corresponding epithelial and soft tissue margins can be combined in the same section.

Soft tissue—treat it as a cube.

cylinder—the anterior and posterior bone margins—should be submitted. Thus, in the case illustrated, the margins taken include anterior, posterior, medial, lateral, and inferior soft tissue margins; anterior, posterior, medial, and lateral epithelial margins; and anterior and posterior bone margins. Obviously, corresponding epithelial and soft tissue margins can be—and, indeed, usually are—included in the same section.

Step 4. Document the Relationship Between Any Lesions and Each Component of the Specimen

All lesions, as well as sections demonstrating the relationship of each lesion to each of the various components of the specimen, should be sampled. For example, in the specimen illustrated, sections should be taken showing the relationship of the tumor to the bone, of the tumor to the surface of the epithelium, and of the tumor to the muscle.

While we find this geometric approach to specimens helpful, you may wish to develop your own system for complex specimens. Whatever approach you choose, remember that your ultimate goal is to provide the clinician with the information needed for the appropriate management of the patient.

7 Radical Neck Dissection

Neck dissections for the en bloc removal of cervical lymph nodes come in a variety of shapes and sizes. The radical neck dissection is the standard procedure to which all other neck dissections are compared. It includes resection of the sternocleidomastoid muscle, the submandibular gland, the internal jugular vein, and the lymph nodes from levels I to V. The goal of the surgical pathologist in evaluating these specimens is simply to identify the number of lymph nodes involved by tumor at each level.

Start by orienting the specimen. The dissection is shaped like a Z. The pink-tan, lobulated submandibular gland is usually easy to identify, and it occupies level I, the most anterosuperior aspect of the specimen. The internal jugular vein, as its name implies, is present on the internal (medial) surface of the sternocleidomastoid muscle. Using these two anatomic landmarks, one can both orient the specimen and determine which side it was taken from. After orienting the specimen, measure its overall dimensions. Next, open the jugular vein along its length, and look for tumor involvement or thrombosis. Sample any abnormality in the vein.

The specimen can now be divided into its five levels and each level separately dissected for lymph nodes. First, dissect off level I, which includes the submandibular salivary gland and the triangle of soft tissues anterior to the sternocleidomastoid muscle. Next, remove level V, the triangle of fatty connective tissue posterior to the muscle. Finally, levels II, III, and IV can be separated off by dividing the sternocleidomastoid muscle into equal thirds. Level II, the upper jugular group, is composed of the lymph nodes around the upper third of the sternocleidomastoid muscle. Level III, the middle jugular group, is composed of the lymph nodes around the middle third of the sternocleidomastoid muscle, and level IV, the lower jugular group, is composed of lymph nodes around the lower third. Now search for the lymph nodes. The best place to look for lymph nodes in each level is in the fatty connective tissue. Lymph nodes usually will not be found within the sternocleidomastoid muscle itself. A representative section of each node, including a designation of the level from which it was taken, should be submitted for histology. Be sure that the section includes the capsule of the lymph node and a rim of the perinodal fat. In addition, the salivary gland in level I should be measured, described, and serially sectioned. If any masses are found in the salivary gland, the gland should be dissected as described in Chapter 5. If no abnormalities are grossly apparent, simply submit a representative section for histology. Finally, representative sections of any tumor involving the sternocleidomastoid muscle or extranodal soft tissue should be submitted for histology. If a group of matted lymph nodes is present, it will be impossible to dissect out each individual lymph node. In these cases, submit two sections through the level involved to document the extensive nature of the tumor.

A number of variations of the radical neck dissection exist. These are well described by Robbins and co-workers.[1] Each of these can be dissected using the same approach outlined above. First, orient the specimen. Without important landmarks (e.g., submandibular gland, internal jugular vein), you will usually have to rely on the surgeon to designate each level. Second, identify the lymph nodes at each level. Third, sample each node for histology.

Submandibular
gland

Internal
jugular
vein

Sternocleidomastoid
muscle

Medial surface of the
right neck

Level I

II

III

IV

Level V

Lateral surface of the
right neck

Radical Neck Dissection

1. Orient the specimen. The salivary gland occupies the most anterosuperior aspect of the resection, and the internal jugular vein lies over the medial surface of the sternocleidomastoid muscle.

2. Open the vein, and sample any lesions.

3. Separate off each level, identify all of the lymph nodes, and sample each node for histology.

4. Examine the salivary gland, and submit a section for histology.

5. Section the muscle, and submit a section of it if any lesions are encountered.

Important Issues to Address in Your Surgical Pathology Report on Radical Neck Dissections

- What procedure was performed, and what structures/organs are present?
- What is the total number of lymph nodes present at each level, and how many of these are involved by tumor?
- Does the carcinoma extend beyond the lymph node and into extranodal soft tissue?
- Is the internal jugular vein thrombosed and/or infiltrated by tumor?
- Do the salivary glands, muscle, and soft tissues contain tumor or any other pathology?

III   The Digestive System

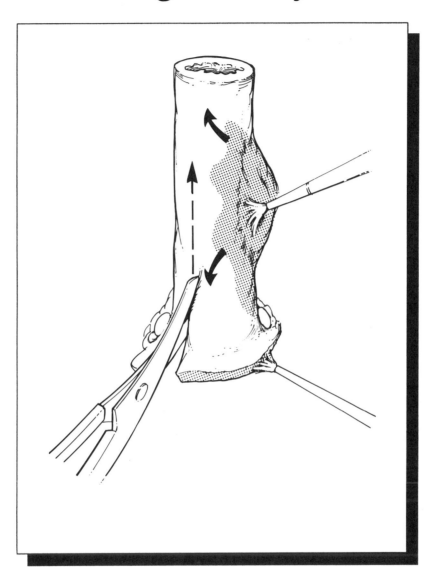

8 Esophagus

Esophagectomies

Esophagectomies are almost always performed to resect neoplastic processes. The nature and extent of the neoplastic process, however, may be quite variable. Lesions may range from microscopic alterations in patients with a long history of Barrett's esophagus to large fungating carcinomas in patients presenting with obstruction and dysphagia.

Esophagectomy specimens are anatomically simples structures consisting essentially of a straight muscular tube. Orientation is seldom difficult, since a cuff of stomach is resected in continuity with the distal portion of esophagus. After measuring the dimensions of the specimen, ink its outer surface and the mucosal margins. The esophagus, you will recall, does not have a serosa. Rather, the surface of the soft tissues investing the esophagus represents a true soft tissue margin.

Next, open the esophagus to expose the mucosal surface. As illustrated, this step involves cutting through the wall of the esophagus from one end of the specimen to the other. A common mistake is to cut directly across the tumor. This can be a costly error, since it distorts the appearance of the tumor and disrupts the tumor's relationship with underlying structures. Fortunately, this can easily be avoided by first localizing the tumor and then cutting through the esophageal wall on the opposite side. The key, of course, is to pay close attention to the location of the tumor before heedlessly wielding the scissors. Begin by palpating the unopened esophagus. Areas of induration often divulge the location and extent of an infiltrating tumor.

Next, cut the esophagus in a stepwise fashion: Inspect the lumen with a probing finger, and then advance the scissors one cautious cut at a time.

Once the specimen is opened, observe the appearance and thickness of the esophageal wall. If strictures are present, measure the luminal circumference of the esophagus at the point of narrowing and at the point of maximal dilatation proximal to the stricture. Carefully inspect the mucosa. If a tumor is not seen, try to identify the site of a previous biopsy. Biopsy site changes can be subtle. Look for focal areas of mucosal hemorrhage, ulceration, scarring, and puckering. Identify the gastroesophageal junction (GEJ), the point at which the tubular esophagus joins the saccular stomach. It is usually located 1 to 2 cm from the proximal edges of the gastric folds. Keep in mind that the GEJ does not always correlate with the squamocolumnar mucosal junction. Rather, the squamocolumnar junction normally may occur anywhere within the distal 2 to 3 cm of esophagus. The gastric mucosa is velvety red, and it contrasts sharply with the smooth gray appearance of the squamous epithelium lining the esophagus. Proximal extension of the squamocolumnar junction beyond the distal 2 to 3 cm of the esophagus is abnormal and suggestive of Barrett's esophagus.

If a tumor is apparent, note its dimensions, its location with respect to the squamocolumnar and gastroesophageal junctions, and the distance of the tumor's edges from the margins of resection. The distance of the tumor to the resection margin should always be measured in the fresh specimen; fixation causes the mucosa to retract, giving the appearance that the muco-

Esophagus

Locate the
tumor before
opening the
esophagus.

Lymph nodes

Proximal
stomach

Ink the soft
tissues overlying
the tumor.

Open the
esophagus on the
side opposite the
tumor.

Proximal
margin

Tumor

Deep
margin

Distal
margin

Squamocolumnar
junction

Esophagectomy

1. Orient the specimen
   using the distal cuff
   of the stomach.

2. Ink the outer surface
   and mucosal mar-
   gins.

3. Palpate the tumor
   with a finger, and
   open the esophagus
   on the side opposite
   the tumor.

4. Examine adherent
   soft tissue for lymph
   nodes.

5. Submit sections of
   the proximal, distal,
   and deep margins;
   the squamocolum-
   nar junction; sec-
   tions of the tumor to
   show its greatest
   depth of invasion;
   and any lymph
   nodes.

sal margins are closer to the tumor than they actually are. Photograph the opened specimen to document the gross findings. Before placing the specimen in formalin, ask yourself if fresh tissue should be submitted for special studies. Pin the specimen flat onto a wax tablet, and submerge it in formalin until well fixed.

Once the specimen is fixed, section through the full thickness of the tumor and the underlying wall to determine the level and depth of tumor extension. Submit at least two full-thickness sections of the esophagus at the level where it appears most deeply penetrated by the tumor. Be sure that these sections include the inked soft tissue surface so that this margin can be assessed. Also take sections of tumor to demonstrate its relationship to the adjacent mucosa, and liberally sample areas of Barrett's mucosa. In those cases where a tumor is not grossly apparent, three specific areas should be entirely submitted for histologic evaluation: (1) the squamocolumnar junction; (2) areas of abnormal mucosa such as the red velvety changes seen in Barrett's mucosa; and (3) previous biopsy sites. Sample the proximal and distal resection margins using perpendicular sections if the tumor is close or shave sections if the tumor is far removed.

Carefully dissect the soft tissues investing the esophagus for lymph nodes. Most of these lymph nodes will be found in the region of the gastroesophageal junction. Submit a representative section of each lymph node found for histologic evaluation.

Important Issues to Address in Your Surgical Pathology Report on Esophagectomies

- What procedure was performed, and what structures/organs are present?
- In which portion of the esophagus does the tumor arise (cervical, upper thoracic, midthoracic, lower thoracic)?
- What are the histologic type and grade of the tumor?
- What are the size, location, and depth of maximum invasion of the tumor? Is it *in situ*? If invasive, into which level does it invade (lamina propria or submucosa, muscularis propria, adventitia, or adjacent structures)?
- Does the tumor involve any resection margins? Specifically, what is the status of the proximal (esophageal), distal (stomach), and deep (adventitial) margins?
- What is the condition of the non-neoplastic/preneoplastic esophagus? For example, are there changes of Barrett's esophagus, dysplasia, inflammation, or infection?
- Is there evidence of metastatic disease? Record the number of lymph nodes examined and the number of lymph node metastases.

9 Stomach

Total and Partial Gastrectomies

Stomach specimens come in a variety of shapes and sizes depending on the pathologic process for which the stomach is removed. For example, a small portion of stomach may be removed for peptic ulcer disease, while the entire stomach and even adjacent organs can be resected when an infiltrating cancer is present. Regardless of the specimen's size and shape, a wise approach is to regard every stomach resection as though it potentially harbors a malignant neoplasm. Do not be betrayed by the innocent-looking ulcer. Instead, take care to evaluate the resection margins, adequately sample the lesion, and diligently search for lymph nodes. With this approach, the dissection should always be adequate, even in that rare instance when a carcinoma is incidentally discovered in a benign-appearing ulcer.

The dissection of a stomach specimen begins with a basic understanding of the stomach's anatomy. This understanding is important for two reasons: First, the anatomic regions of the stomach are functionally and histologically distinct; thus, each region of the stomach should be individually assessed. Second, anatomic landmarks can be used to orient most stomach specimens. The four divisions of the stomach are the cardia, fundus, body, and antrum. The cardia is the rim of the stomach that surrounds the gastroesophageal junction (GEJ). The fundus is the dome-shaped region of the stomach that sweeps superior to the GEJ. The body accounts for the major portion of the stomach. It narrows distally as it merges with the antrum.

The antrum is the distal third of the stomach and includes the pyloric sphincter. The anatomic boundaries separating these regions are not distinct, at least not in the unopened specimen. Once the mucosal surface is exposed, however, the demarcation between the body and antrum can be easier to appreciate. For example, the body shows prominent rugal folds, whereas the mucosa of the antrum is comparatively flat. This flattened antral surface forms a V. The nadir of the V rests on the lesser curvature and points toward the proximal portion of the stomach. Other landmarks that are useful in orienting the specimen include the greater curvature, the broad and convex inferior aspect of the stomach; the lesser curvature, the concave superior aspect of the stomach; and the pyloric ring, a thick muscular collar at the outlet of the stomach. In more limited stomach resections, these landmarks may not be present and correct orientation relies upon the surgeon's designation.

Begin your examination by clearly marking the stomach resection margins. Keep in mind that these margins may be difficult to reconstruct once the specimen has been opened. One simple method is to ink the margins and then place four safety pins—two on either side of the greater curvature at both the proximal and distal margins. By cutting the specimen between these safety pins, you can easily reconstruct the opened specimen simply by juxtaposing the two pins.

To facilitate handling of the stomach, remove the bulky omenta (when present) suspended from the greater and lesser curvatures of the stomach. Do not discard this fat. Instead, set it

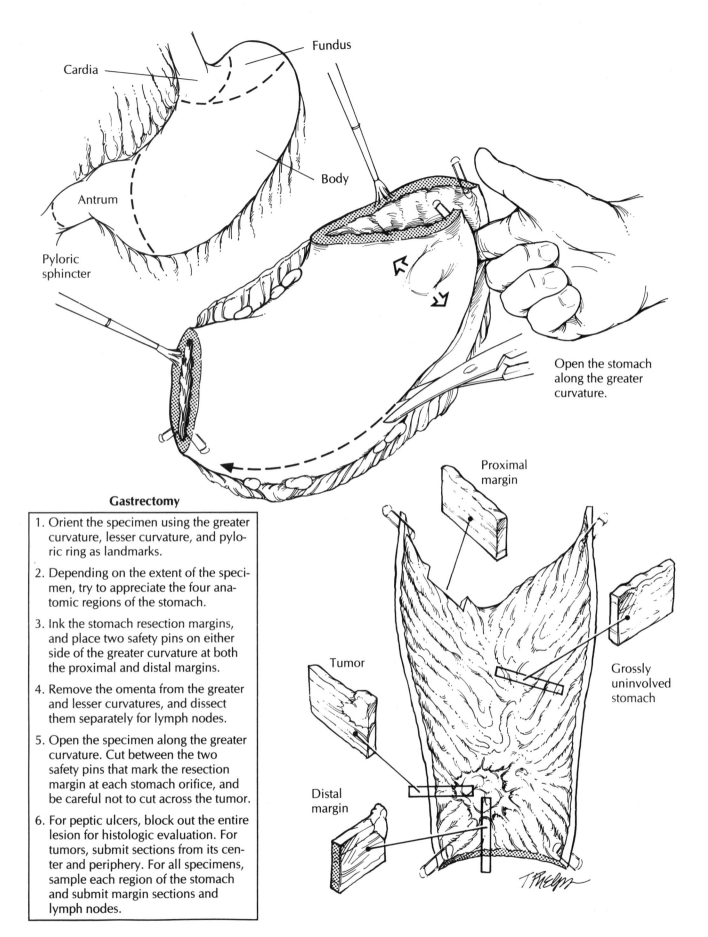

Cardia

Fundus

Body

Antrum

Pyloric sphincter

Open the stomach along the greater curvature.

Proximal margin

Grossly uninvolved stomach

Tumor

Distal margin

T. Phelan

Gastrectomy

1. Orient the specimen using the greater curvature, lesser curvature, and pyloric ring as landmarks.

2. Depending on the extent of the specimen, try to appreciate the four anatomic regions of the stomach.

3. Ink the stomach resection margins, and place two safety pins on either side of the greater curvature at both the proximal and distal margins.

4. Remove the omenta from the greater and lesser curvatures, and dissect them separately for lymph nodes.

5. Open the specimen along the greater curvature. Cut between the two safety pins that mark the resection margin at each stomach orifice, and be careful not to cut across the tumor.

6. For peptic ulcers, block out the entire lesion for histologic evaluation. For tumors, submit sections from its center and periphery. For all specimens, sample each region of the stomach and submit margin sections and lymph nodes.

49

aside for later dissection. Next, open the stomach along its entire length, cutting between the safety pins at each stomach orifice. To avoid cutting across the lesion, insert a probing finger into the lumen, and explore the inner surface of the stomach ahead of the advancing scissors. Be flexible in your approach. Whenever possible, cut along the greater curvature, but always be ready to tailor the dissection to avoid cutting through a tumor. When the line of excision along the greater curvature is obstructed by a tumor, the lesser curvature may serve as an alternative route for opening the stomach.

Once the stomach is opened, evaluate each of the three layers of the stomach—the mucosa, wall, and serosa. Do the gastric folds appear thickened or effaced? Assess the number, size, location, and appearance of any lesions. For ulcerative lesions, carefully note those features that are helpful in distinguishing benign ulcers (e.g., sharply defined margins, smooth and flat borders, straight walls, clean base) from gastric carcinomas (e.g., irregular margins, thickened and heaped-up borders, shaggy base). Important measurements include not only the dimensions of the lesion but also the distance from the lesion to the resection margins. This distance, known as the *gross clearance*, should be measured while the specimen is fresh, because the mucosa tends to retract during fixation. Photography plays an important role in the evaluation of stomach specimens. Sections taken for histology can be mapped with considerable detail on a Polaroid photograph of the specimen. This is a useful method for correlating the histologic features with the anatomic region of the stomach. Next, examine and describe the wall and the serosa of the stomach. Are any mural nodules noted? Is the wall diffusely thickened or focally indurated? Are any serosal lesions noted? Is the serosa retracted? Collect fresh tissue samples for special studies as needed, then pin the specimen flat on a wax tablet, and submerge it in formalin until well fixed.

"Better safe than sorry" is a wise policy when sampling the stomach. Consider again the prudence of viewing each lesion with the suspicion that it represents a malignant neoplasm. Thoroughly sample all lesions, evaluate every margin, and diligently search for lymph nodes. For lesions that are clinically believed to be peptic ulcers, submit the entire ulcer in a sequential fashion so that an underlying malignancy is not missed. When a tumor is apparent, section through it to determine whether it extends into or through the stomach wall. Submit sections from the center of the tumor to determine its maximum depth of invasion. Also submit sections from the tumor's periphery to demonstrate the transition between the tumor and the adjacent gastric mucosa. When the stomach appears diffusely thickened by an infiltrative process (e.g., linitis plastica) submit sections from all four regions of the stomach. Margins should generally be sampled using perpendicular sections when the tumor is close, and shave sections when the tumor is far removed. Submit a representative section of all lymph nodes. Keep the greater and lesser omental node groups separate. A good place to find lymph nodes is at the point where the omenta attach to the stomach.

The grossly uninvolved stomach should also be sampled for histologic evaluation. Depending on the extent of the resection, these sections should represent all four regions of the stomach, the squamocolumnar junction, and if present, the contiguous esophagus. For extended resections that include adjacent colon, spleen, liver, and/or pancreas, sections should be taken to determine the presence of direct tumor extension, tumor metastases, and the adequacy of surgical excision (i.e., the status of the margins).

Important Issues to Address in Your Surgical Pathology Report on Gastrectomies

- What procedure was performed, and what structures/organs are present?
- What are the location (cardia, fundus, body, or antrum), size, type, and histologic grade of the neoplasm?
- What is the extent of the neoplasm? Specify into which level of the wall of the stomach the tumor invades (e.g., mucosa, submucosa, muscularis propria, subserosal soft tissues, or serosa). Does the tumor extend beyond the serosa to involve adjacent structures?
- Does the tumor involve the soft tissue and/or mucosal margins? What is the distance of the mucosal margin from the edge of the tumor?
- What is the condition of the non-neoplastic

stomach (e.g., changes of gastritis or presence of intestinal metaplasia or ulceration)?

• Is there evidence of metastatic disease? Record the number of lymph nodes examined and the number of lymph node metastases. Also document if any metastases are to lymph nodes located more than 3 cm from the edge of the tumor.

10 Non-neoplastic Intestinal Disease

Small Biopsies

Proper tissue orientation is a critical part of the histologic evaluation of biopsies of the gastrointestinal tract. Tissue orientation is a two-step process that involves the coordinated actions of the endoscopist and the histotechnologist. The endoscopist should mount the biopsy mucosal side up on an appropriate solid surface (e.g., filter paper) and place it in fixative. This first step should be done immediately, in the endoscopy suite, so that the specimen does not dry out en route to the surgical pathology laboratory. The histotechnologist can then embed and cut the biopsy specimen perpendicular to the mounting surface. If the specimen is free floating, great care must be taken to identify the mucosal surface for proper embedding. Multiple sections should be cut from each tissue block for histologic evaluation. Step sections are preferred to serial sections so that intervening unstained sections are available for special stains as needed.

Resections of Small and Large Intestine for Inflammatory Bowel Disease

Given the structural simplicity of the intestinal tract and the ease with which the bowel can be opened, there is a strong tendency to rush into these dissections without thinking ahead. The approach to the non-neoplastic bowel specimen requires an effective strategy that gives careful consideration to an organized gross description, specimen photography and fixation, and details of dissection and tissue sampling.

The Organized Gross Description

A good gross description not only describes all the relevant gross findings but presents these findings in an organized fashion. This can be a difficult task in bowel resections, where the specimen may consist of more than one structure (e.g., ileum, appendix, cecum, and colon). Organize your gross description. First, describe the specimen after it has been fixed, examined, and at least partially dissected. This will make it possible to collect all of the gross findings and integrate them into an organized statement. Second, always describe each component of the resection as an individual unit. For example, describe the mucosa, wall, and serosa of the ileum and then move on to the appendix, cecum, and finally the colon. Third, focus on the mucosa. Begin by describing the distribution of mucosal alterations (e.g., diffuse, discontinuous, etc.) and then describe the specific characteristics of these changes (e.g., ulcerated, granular, etc.). Of course, no gross description is complete without a description of the wall, serosa, and mesentery; but for inflammatory bowel disease, a less detailed description of these layers will generally suffice.

Specimen Dissection

Given the structural simplicity of the bowel, opening these specimens is generally straight-

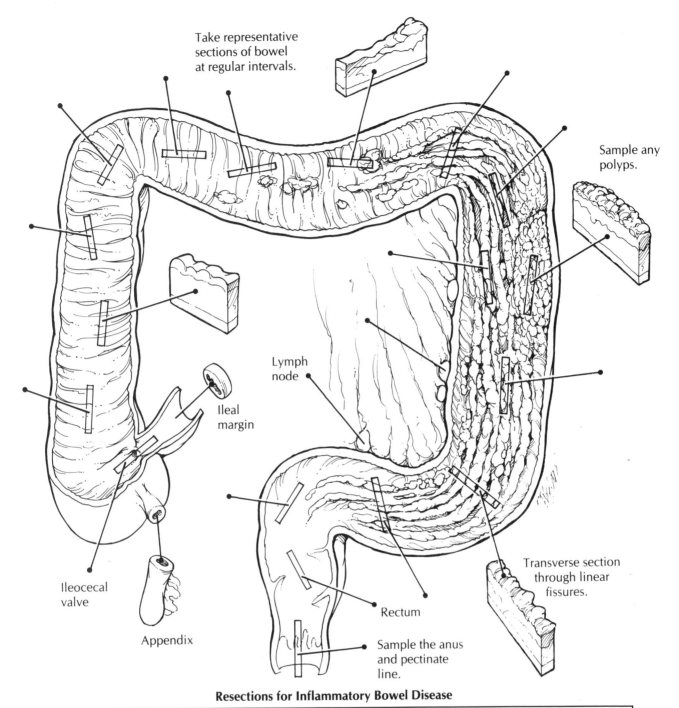

Take representative sections of bowel at regular intervals.

Sample any polyps.

Lymph node

Ileal margin

Ileocecal valve

Appendix

Rectum

Sample the anus and pectinate line.

Transverse section through linear fissures.

Resections for Inflammatory Bowel Disease

1. Orient the specimen. The large intestine can be distinguished from the small intestine by its larger diameter and by the presence of longitudinal muscle bands, sacculations, and the appendices epiploicae.

2. Identify and measure all components of the specimen (do not forget to look for the appendix).

3. Remove the mesentery. Open the small bowel along its mesenteric border, and the large bowel along the anterior teniae coli. Rinse the bowel, pin it flat on a cork or wax tablet, and submerge it in formalin until well fixed.

4. Describe the specimen in a systematic fashion. Include a description of the mucosa, wall, and serosa of each component of the specimen.

5. Sample all areas of the bowel by submitting sections at regular 10-cm intervals. Also include sections of the appendix, ileocecal valve, margins, mesenteric vessels, any focal lesions, and representative lymph nodes from all regions of the bowel.

forward. When possible, the small intestine should be opened adjacent to the mesentery. In contrast, the large intestine should be opened on the antimesenteric border along the anterior (free) teniae coli. Remove the mesentery before fixing the bowel. Treat the mesenteric soft tissues as though a carcinoma will be discovered in the bowel resection, keeping in mind that carcinomas may arise in the setting of long-standing inflammatory bowel disease. For total colectomies, remove the mesentery as six separate portions, and designate these as proximal ascending, distal ascending, proximal transverse, distal transverse, proximal descending, and distal descending. Although only representative lymph nodes need to be submitted, the six portions should be clearly labeled and saved for easy retrieval if more extensive lymph node sampling is later required.

Specimen Fixation

The bowel should be fixed before it is photographed, described, and sectioned. Subtle mucosal alterations (e.g., erosions, ulcerations, areas of hemorrhage, etc.) that may not be apparent in the fresh specimen are often well defined once the specimen is fixed. In most cases, the specimen can be opened and pinned on a solid surface as a flat sheet and then submerged in formalin. Some specimens may be so distorted that they cannot be easily opened and pinned flat without the risk of cutting across structures (e.g., fistulas, diverticuli, etc.) and disrupting important relationships. These distorted specimens may be best handled by infusing formalin into the lumen of the bowel and then clamping both ends of the specimen. Whether the bowel is submerged or infused, fecal material should first be rinsed from the mucosal surface (a more formidable challenge in the unopened specimen) using a gentle stream of an isotonic solution.

Specimen Photography

Photographs of the specimen should be liberally taken to document further the gross findings, especially the distribution and nature of the mucosal alterations. Photograph the specimen after it has been opened and fixed. Photographs of the unopened bowel are generally useless. Fixation tends to both accentuate the mucosal alterations and reduce the amount of reflected light. Always position the specimen anatomically on the photography table. Total colectomies, for example, should be positioned so that the ascending colon is to the anatomic right, the descending colon is to the left, and the transverse colon is to the top and center. Finally, include close-up photographs to illustrate the details of the mucosal pathology.

Tissue Sampling

To evaluate the distribution of inflammatory changes in the specimen, all areas of the bowel should be sampled for histologic evaluation. One method that consistently ensures adequate sampling is to submit representative sections at 10-cm intervals, beginning at the proximal end of the specimen and proceeding distally in a step-wise fashion. This not only will ensure that the mucosa is well sampled, but will also provide information on the distribution of the disease process. Of course, sections of any focal lesions such as ulcers or polyps should be submitted in addition to these interval sections. Sections should also be taken of the appendix and the ileocecal valve when these structures are present. When no tumor is grossly apparent, the resection margins may be taken as shave sections. In addition to sampling the mesentery for lymph nodes, submit sections of mesenteric blood vessels and of any focal lesions such as fistula tracts or areas of fat necrosis. Sketch the site from which all sections were taken on the Polaroid photograph with a permanent waterproof marker. Take longitudinal sections (i.e., parallel to the teniae coli). Exceptions are permitted when, for example, a linear ulcer is best demonstrated by a transverse section through the bowel.

Once these principles regarding gross description, fixation, dissections, and sampling are mastered, the inflammatory bowel specimen can be handled with relative ease. The initial step is to identify the structures that are present in the resected specimen. The large intestine is readily distinguished from the small intestine by its larger diameter and the presence of longitudinal muscle bands (the teniae coli), sacculations (the haustra), and the appendices epiploicae. In addition, the small intestine shows mucosal folds that stretch across the entire circumference of the bowel, whereas the mucosal folds of the large intestine are discontinuous. Several features may be helpful in appreciating the various regions of the large intestine. The cecum is usually quite apparent, and it can be used to identify the origin of the ascending colon. The transverse colon can be recognized by its large mesenteric pedicle attachment, while the sigmoid colon has a relatively short mesenteric pedicle. When a portion of rectum is included in the specimen, it can be distinguished from the sigmoid colon by the absence of a peritoneal surface lining.

The initial description should be limited to a list of the structures present and the dimensions of each. Further handling of the bowel is facilitated by removing the mesenteric fat. As described previously, these soft tissues should be removed according to their anatomic location, and each portion should be clearly labeled so that is can be easily identified and retrieved. Most prosectors have an easier time finding mesenteric lymph nodes while these tissues are still in the fresh state. Remember, most of the lymph nodes are found at the junction of the bowel and mesenteric fat. Open the bowel along its entire length, cutting the small bowel along its mesenteric attachment and the large along the anterior teniae. Gently rinse any fecal material from the mucosal surface using a stream of isotonic solution. Pin the opened bowel flat on a solid surface, and submerge it in formalin.

Once the specimen is fixed, complete the examination of the mucosa, noting in the gross description the distribution and characteristic of the mucosal alterations. Place the bowel in its correct anatomic position, and photograph it. Take a Polaroid photograph of the entire specimen, so that the sites from which histologic sections were taken can be marked on the picture, and take close-up views of focal lesions.

Remember to section all regions of the bowel by using a method of stepwise sectioning at regular (i.e., 10-cm) intervals. Specific bowel sections should include the proximal and distal resection margins, the ileocecal valve, the appendix, and any focal lesions. If a neoplasm is not found, sampling of representative lymph nodes from each level will suffice. Sampling of the mesentery should also include a section of the mesenteric blood vessels and sections of any focal lesions.

Important Issues to Address in Your Surgical Pathology Report on Non-neoplastic Intestinal Disease

- What procedure was performed, and what structures/organs are present?
- What disease processes are present, and what is their location?
- For inflammatory processes, are any diverticuli, strictures, fistulas, or perforations present?
- Does the mucosa show any preneoplastic or neoplastic changes? (See Chapter 11).
- Do the lymph nodes show any evidence of an inflammatory process or metastatic disease? Record the number of lymph nodes examined and the presence or absence of lymph node metastases.
- What is the status of the mesenteric vessels?

11 Neoplastic Intestinal Disease

Polypectomies

Polyps of the gastrointestinal tract are usually removed endoscopically by a single incision at the base of the polyp stalk. Although these specimens lack the size and complexity of more extended bowel resections, they are delicate structures that require meticulous processing. First, obtain relevant clinical information such as the patient's history, the endoscopic findings, and the anatomic site from which the polyp was removed. Next, turn your attention to the specimen itself. The polypectomy specimen poses three important questions to the surgical pathologist: (1) Are adenomatous changes present? (2) Is infiltrating carcinoma present, and if it is, does it infiltrate into the stalk? (3) Do any of the neoplastic changes extend to the resection margin at the base of the stalk? Clearly, the polypectomy specimen must be carefully oriented and processed so that these issues can be addressed.

The key to orienting the polyp is to find its stalk. This may require careful inspection, since a short stalk is often overshadowed by the much larger head of the polyp. After finding the stalk, mark its base (i.e., the resection margin) with either ink or colored tattoo powder. Measure the height and diameter of the polyp. Next, place the specimen in formalin for fixation. Given the soft and spongy consistency of the fresh polyp, sectioning of the polyp is greatly facilitated if it is well fixed.

Once fixed, the specimen should be sectioned in a way to show the relationship of the stalk to the head of the polyp. As illustrated, this relationship is usually best demonstrated by tri-secting the polyp into two lateral caps and one median section that includes the stalk and the center of the head. The median section should demonstrate the largest cross-sectional area of the head of the polyp, its interface with the stalk, and the surgical margin. The importance of trisecting the polyp is readily apparent if one pauses to considers the impact of this method on the histologic sections. Serial sections into the median section of a trisected polyp will approach the point of interest, the center of the polyp. To avoid missing a small focus of carcinoma, submit the entire specimen for histologic evaluation.

Important Issues to Address in your Surgical Pathology Report on Polyps

- What procedure was performed, and what structures/organs are present?
- What is the histologic type of the polyp (e.g., adenomatous, hyperplastic, hamartomatous, inflammatory, etc.)?
- For adenomatous polyps, is the polyp architecturally tubular, villous, or tubulovillous, and what is the histologic grade of the neoplasm?
- If a carcinoma is present, what is the depth of invasion of the tumor? (Specify the presence or absence of invasion of the stalk and of the submucosa at the base of the stalk or base of a sessile polyp.)
- Is there evidence of vascular invasion?
- What is the status of the resection margin at the base? Does the adenomatous epithelium or the infiltrating carcinoma extend to this margin?

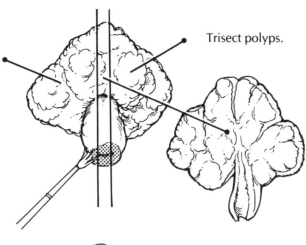

Trisect polyps.

Resections of Intestinal Neoplasms

1. Orient the specimen. Record its length and diameter proximal and distal to the tumor. Describe the serosa.
2. Open the bowel on the side opposite the tumor. Record the size of the tumor and the distance to each margin. Section the tumor, and document its deepest gross penetration.
3. Remove the mesentery, and submit representative sections of each node by level. Look for vascular invasion.
4. Submit sections of tumor to demonstrate its deepest penetration and relationship to normal mucosa. Submit sections of the proximal and distal margins, other lesions, normal mucosa, all lymph nodes, and any attached structures or organs.

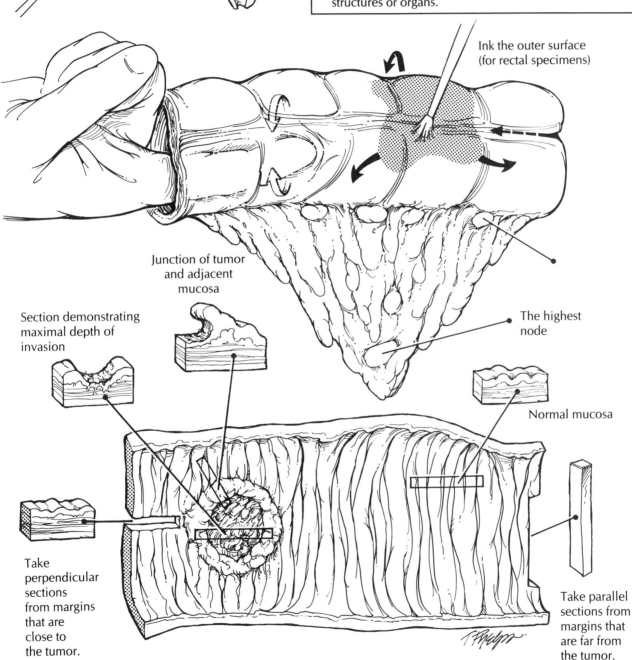

Ink the outer surface
(for rectal specimens)

Junction of tumor
and adjacent
mucosa

Section demonstrating
maximal depth of
invasion

The highest
node

Normal mucosa

Take
perpendicular
sections
from margins
that are
close to
the tumor.

Take parallel
sections from
margins that
are far from
the tumor.

Resections of Intestinal Neoplasms

The pathologic evaluation of resected intestinal neoplasms plays an integral part in determining the patient's prognosis and in selecting the appropriate primary or adjuvant therapy. As is true for other specimens, a systematic approach to your dissection is the best way to ensure that all of the appropriate information is included in your final report.

Start with the patient's history. This should include both the patient's clinical history (Crohn's disease, ulcerative colitis, polyps, family history) and the relevant endoscopic findings. Next, identify the segment of bowel that was resected, and orient the specimen. As described in Chapter 10, the large intestine is readily distinguished from the small intestine by its larger diameter and the presence of longitudinal muscle bands (the teniae coli), sacculations (the haustra), and the appendices epiploicae. In addition, the small intestine shows mucosal folds that stretch across the entire circumference of the bowel, whereas the large intestinal mucosal folds are discontinuous. The rectum can be distinguished from the colon by the absence of a peritoneal surface covering the rectum. Record the length and the diameter of the bowel. The diameter should be recorded both proximal and distal to any lesions. Look for and document the presence and appearance of any other structures, such as the appendix. Next, describe the serosa. Are any diverticula, gross perforations, or serosal nodules present?

As noted above, the rectum lacks a serosal lining. Therefore, the outer surface of the rectum represents a true soft tissue margin, and these soft tissues should be inked. Otherwise, only the proximal and distal margins need to be inked. When opening the bowel, make every effort not to cut through the tumor. First, localize the tumor by palpating the specimen and probing the lumen of the bowel with your finger, then open the bowel on the side opposite the tumor. If a tumor cannot be appreciated

grossly, simply open the small intestine adjacent to the mesentery, the colon along the anterior (free) teniae, and the rectum along the midline anteriorly. Once the specimen has been opened, gently rinse off the intestinal contents using a stream of isotonic saline.

Next, systematically describe the opened specimen. Start with the tumor. Document its location relative to the margins and to any landmarks, such as the ileocecal valve or the pectinate line. Describe the size of the tumor in its longitudinal and transverse dimensions, as well at its gross configuration (endophytic, pedunculated, sessile, diffusely infiltrative, or annular). Multiple cancers should be looked for, described and labeled separately. After the tumor has been described, make multiple parallel 2-3-mm sections through the tumor, and note its deepest gross penetration. Also note the distance from the tumor to the soft tissue or *radial margin*. This is the distance from the outermost part of the tumor to the lateral margin of resection along a radius drawn from the center of the lumen of the bowel through the deepest penetration of the tumor. The soft tissue margin is only important for rectal cancers and for colon cancers located on the mesenteric aspect of the bowel.

After the tumor has been described, turn your attention to the remainder of the bowel. Be systematic in your description. For example, begin with the mucosa, wall, and serosa of the proximal portion of the specimen and then proceed distally. When describing the mucosa, note diverticuli, changes of inflammatory bowel disease, polyps, and ischemic changes. A systematic approach to your gross dictation will ensure that all important findings are included.

We like to examine the soft tissues for lymph nodes in the fresh state because the nodes are easier to palpate and because they retain their pink color, which contrasts to the yellow fat. The next step, therefore, is to dissect the mesentery. Look for and sample any lymph nodes adjacent to the point of ligation of the vascular pedicle, and designate these as the highest lymph nodes. Next, cut the mesentery close to the bowel, maintaining anatomic orientation. Do not remove any areas in which the subserosal soft tissues are involved by tumor. Sample these as a part of the deep margin after the specimen has been fixed. Then divide the detached mesenteric fat into groups: those proximal to the tumor, those at the level of the tumor, and those distal to the tumor. If any great vessels are present, identify and separately designate the nodes adjacent to them. Thinly section the mesenteric fat at each level, and examine and palpate each section for lymph nodes. Submit for histology a representative section of each identified node. When looking for the nodes, remember that they are frequently present at the junction of the bowel wall and the mesentery. When submitting the lymph nodes for histologic processing, remember to designate the level from which they were taken. Also examine the veins and arteries in the mesentery for tumors or thrombi. If any are present, submit a representative section of the involved vessel for histologic examination. After the mesentery has been examined, separately bundle each level in labeled paper towels with rubber bands for storage. Should you ever have to return to the mesentery, the orientation will be preserved. The specimen can now be pinned to a wax tablet and fixed overnight.

After the specimen is well fixed, it can be sampled. Start with the tumor. Submit at least two sections: one from the edge of the tumor to show the junction of tumor and normal bowel, and one from the point of deepest tumor penetration into the wall of the bowel. If the tumor does not grossly appear to involve the bowel wall, then submit the entire base of the lesion to demonstrate the presence or absence of invasion. Submit the proximal and distal margins. If the tumor is close to a margin, these sections should be perpendicular (longitudinal), and if the tumor is far from a margin, these sections can be parallel (transverse). Next, sample any other lesions. When sampling polyps, remember to include both the head and stalk in your

sections. Submit representative sections of normal bowel mucosa and wall, and submit representative sections of all remaining structures/organs, such as the appendix and terminal ileum. Remember that longitudinal sections are better than transverse sections when sampling the colon wall.

Important Issues to Address in Your Surgical Pathology Report on Resections for Intestinal Neoplasms*

- What procedure was performed, and what structures/organs are present?
- What is the location of the tumor?
- What are the dimensions of the tumor?
- What is the gross configuration of the tumor (endophytic, pedunculated, sessile, diffusely infiltrating, annular)?
- What are the histologic type and grade of the neoplasm?
- What is the maximum depth of invasion of the tumor? Is it *in situ*, or does it extend into the lamina propria, submucosa, muscularis propria, or through the muscularis propria into subserosa? Does the tumor extend into other organs, or does it perforate into the visceral peritoneum?
- Is any vascular invasion identified?
- What is the status of the margins (proximal, distal, and radial)?
- How many lymph node metastases were identified, and how many lymph nodes were sampled at each level?
- Are any other lesions noted (e.g., adenomas, intestinal inflammatory disease, dysplasia, etc.)?

---

*Adapted from Henson DE, Hutter RVP, Sobin LH, Bowman HE. Protocol for the examination for specimens removed from patients with colorectal cancer. *Arch Pathol Lab Med.* 1994;118:122–125.

12 Appendix

Simple Appendectomies

The appendix is a common specimen in the surgical pathology laboratory. The dissection of these specimens is not complex, since most appendectomies are performed for simple acute appendicitis. Even so, the appendix is all too often not examined appropriately. Cursory examination of the appendix is a pitfall to be avoided. Instead, develop the habit of thoroughly examining every appendix. Regard every appendiceal specimen as an opportunity to uncover unsuspected pathologic processes.

The major objectives in dissecting the simple appendectomy specimen are to document the presence or absence of inflammation and to search for incidental neoplasms. These objectives are met by examining each component of the appendix—the serosa, wall, mucosa, and lumen—in a sequential manner. Begin by inspecting the outer surface of the appendix and the attached mesoappendix. Inflammatory processes often convert the glistening, smooth, tan serosa into a surface that is dull, shaggy, and discolored. Carefully look for perforations. Small transmural perforations that are not easily seen can sometimes be demonstrated by gently infusing formalin into the lumen of the appendix using a syringe. Document the dimensions of the specimen, and then section the appendix so that the wall, the mucosa, and the lumen can be evaluated. As illustrated, bread-loaf the body of the appendix using thin transverse sections, and bivalve the distal 2-cm tip of the appendix using a longitudinal section. Inspect the wall for masses, strictures, edema, and other inflammatory changes. Finally, evaluate the mucosa and the luminal contents for fecaliths, pus, and collec-tions of mucus. If a neoplasm is present, submit a shave margin from the base of the appendix, and be sure to document the size of the tumor, the distance from the tumor to the surgical margin, and the layers of the appendix that are involved. When the lumen is obstructed, attempt to identify the nature of the obstruction, keeping in mind that most tumors of the appendix are discovered in specimens resected for other reasons.

Sections for histologic evaluation should include a transverse section through the base and body and a longitudinal section of the tip. Include a portion of the attached mesoappendix. For a normal-appearing appendix removed by incidental appendectomy, one section from base, body, and tip placed into a single tissue cassette will suffice. For an inflamed appendix, additional sections may be required to demonstrate points of perforation or luminal obstruction. If a mass or mucocele is present, the entire appendix should be submitted in a sequential fashion. The most proximal section from the base of the appendix represents the margin of resection.

Important Issues to Address in Your Surgical Pathology Report on Appendectomies

- What procedure was performed, and what structures/organs are present?
- What are the nature and extent of any inflammatory processes present (e.g., acute appendicitis, abscess formation, gangrene, etc.)? Be sure to mention the presence or absence of perforations and peritonitis.
- What are the type, grade, size, location, and extent of any incidental neoplasms identified? Is the tumor present at the resection margin?

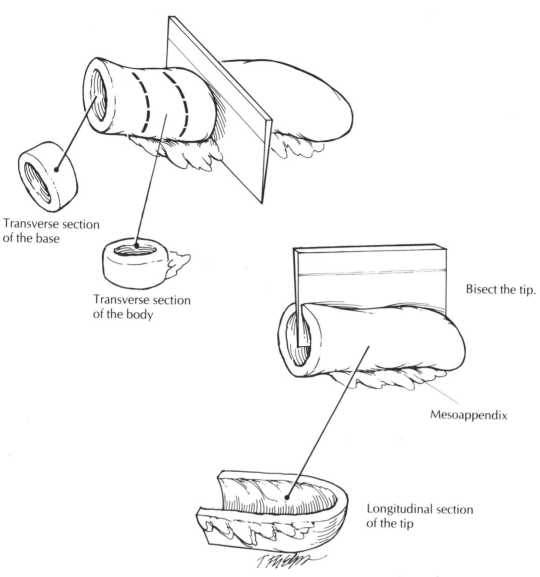

Transverse section
of the base

Transverse section
of the body

Bisect the tip.

Mesoappendix

Longitudinal section
of the tip

Appendectomy

1. Orient and measure the appendix. Carefully look for perforations.

2. Serially section the body of the appendix using transverse sections. Bivalve the tip using a longitudinal section.

3. Describe and measure any tumors.

4. Submit sections of the base, body, and tip of the appendix for histologic evaluation. The entire appendix should be submitted for all tumors and mucoceles.

13 Liver

Biopsies

Biopsies of the liver come in two forms: the delicate needle-core biopsy and the larger wedge biopsy. In either case, the specimen should be measured and submitted in its entirety for routine histology. Thin-core biopsies are particularly susceptible to desiccation. Therefore, unless special studies are indicated, biopsies should be placed in fixative in the operating room. The core biopsy can be embedded whole, while the wedge biopsy may be thick enough to warrant sectioning before submitting to the histology laboratory. When sectioning the wedge biopsy, identify the smooth capsule, and then cut the liver at 0.2-cm intervals perpendicular to this surface. Multiple slides should be prepared from each tissue block for histologic evaluation. Step sections are preferred to serial sections so that the intervening sections are available for special stains. If a storage disease is suspected, then a small portion of the biopsy should be placed in glutaraldehyde for electron microscopy.

Partial Hepatectomy

Focal nodules in the liver can be removed by partial liver resections. The extent of these resections varies from small wedges to the removal of an entire lobe. Regardless of its size, the partial liver resection is not structurally complex. Typically, it consists of a focal lesion surrounded by a variable rim of non-neoplastic liver parenchyma. Several faces of the specimen are covered by a peritoneal lining, but at least one surface shows exposed hepatic paren-

chyma. This exposed surface is the surgical resection margin. This margin has to be correctly identified and oriented. Identification of the resection margin is seldom problematic. Unlike the smooth contour of the peritoneal-lined liver capsule, the resection plane exposes liver parenchyma—which may be fragmented or bloody—and shows cautery effect. On the other hand, orientation of the margin can be very difficult, given the paucity of anatomic landmarks in these limited resections. If the surgeon needs to know the precise location at which a tumor involves or approaches the surgical margin, orientation will require the surgeon's assistance.

Once the margin is identified and the specimen oriented, weigh the specimen, and measure it in each dimension. Examine its contours and surfaces. A bulge in the surface of the liver and/or retraction of the serosa can help localize an intraparenchymal mass. Livers resected for traumatic ruptures should be carefully examined for lacerations of the capsule. Next, rinse the blood from the cut margin, blot it with paper towels, and then ink the dry resection margin. As illustrated, serially section the liver perpendicular to the resection margin. The initial section should pass through the center of the tumor to demonstrate the closest approach of the tumor to the resection margin. Continue sectioning the liver parallel to this first cut at thin (e.g., 0.5-cm) intervals. Examine all cut surfaces for additional nodules.

Record the number, size, location, color, consistency, and circumscription of all lesions. Note the presence or absence of necrosis, hemorrhage, and scarring. Measure the distance from all lesions to the surgical resection margin. If intrahepatic blood vessels are apparent, ex-

Take sections
perpendicular to
the parenchymal margin.

Partial Hepatectomy

1. Weigh and measure the specimen.

2. Identify and ink the liver resection margin.

3. Serially section the liver perpendicular to the resection margin at 0.5-cm intervals.

4. Document the distance from the resection margin to the edge of the tumor.

5. For metastatic lesions, submit sections from the periphery of the tumor and of the margin. Sample primary liver tumors more extensively, including perpendicular sections from the resection margin at points most closely approached by tumor. Representative sections of non-neoplastic liver should also be submitted.

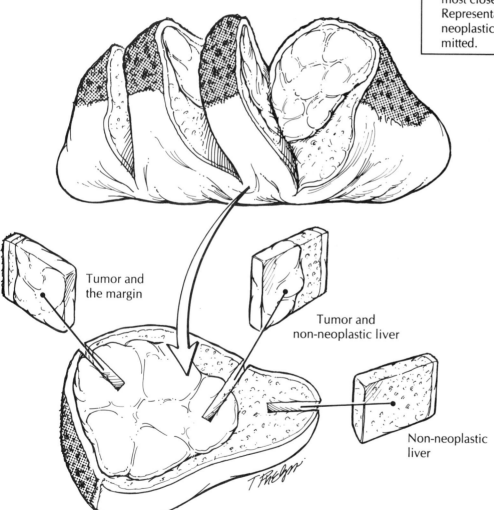

Tumor and
the margin

Tumor and
non-neoplastic liver

Non-neoplastic
liver

Left lobe

Right lobe

Falciform
ligament

Gallbladder

Total Hepatectomy

1. Orient the liver by identifying the four lobes: right, left, caudate, and quadrate. Weigh and measure the liver.

2. Identify and sample the structures of the porta hepatis.

3. Dissect the gallbladder from its bed, and routinely process.

4. Section the liver along its longest axis on either side of the hilum. Serially section the detached portions of the liver perpendicular to the long axis.

5. Submit shave margin sections from the bile duct, hepatic artery and portal vein. Submit three sections each from the right and left lobes, and one section each from the caudate and quadrate lobes. Include standard gallbladder sections.

Quadrate lobe

Inferior
vena cava

Caudate lobe

Shave sections of
bile duct,
hepatic artery, and
portal vein (the
porta hepatis)

amine them for tumor thrombi. Remember to describe the appearance of the non-neoplastic hepatic parenchyma. Is the lesion arising in a background of cirrhosis? Is there intraparenchymal hemorrhage associated with an overlying laceration of the capsule?

Sections of tumors should be taken to demonstrate the relationship of tumor to the surrounding liver parenchyma and of the tumor to the resection margin. Sections from the periphery of the tumor are generally much more informative than are those from the center of the tumor. The periphery of a tumor demonstrates the interface with adjacent tissues, and the periphery of a tumor is often less necrotic than the center. Sample the resection margin using perpendicular sections from the areas closest to the edge of the tumor. Depending on the extent of the resection, several representative sections of the non-neoplastic liver parenchyma should also be submitted for histologic evaluation. These sections of uninvolved liver parenchyma are generally more informative when taken far from the nodule.

Important Issues to Address in Your Surgical Pathology Report on Partial Hepatectomies

- What procedure was performed, and what structures/organs are present?
- How many tumor nodules are present? What are their sizes? Are they confined to one lobe?
- What are the type and histologic grade of the neoplasm? Is the tumor of liver origin or a metastasis from another site?
- Is vascular invasion identified?
- Is the surgical margin involved by tumor? If not, what is the distance from the margin to the edge of the tumor?
- What is the condition of the non-neoplastic liver? Is the non-neoplastic liver cirrhotic? Is there evidence of hepatitis?

Liver Explants

Entire liver resections are encountered in hospitals where liver transplantations are performed. The aim of these dissections is to document the cause of the patient's hepatic failure and, in the cases of liver tumors, to stage the tumor and assess the margins at the porta hepatis. Not infrequently, the cause of the hepatic failure is infectious. Be very careful in handling these specimens, and as always, strictly observe universal precautions. It is not unreasonable to cut several deep sections into the liver parenchyma and then submerge the entire specimen in formalin before further processing.

To sample all regions of the liver adequately and to evaluate the important structures of the porta hepatis, you will need to remember the basic anatomy of the liver. As illustrated, the liver is made up of four lobes. Viewed from above, the right and left lobes are separated by the falciform ligament. The two central lobes are best appreciated by examining the undersurface of the liver. The caudate lobe sits between the portal vein and the inferior vena cava. The quadrate lobe is separated from the right lobe by the gallbladder fossa, from the left lobe by the ligamentum teres, and from the caudate lobe by the portal vein. The major structures forming the porta hepatis are the bile duct, hepatic artery, and portal vein. These three structures maintain a consistent relationship one to another. The duct is most anterior and to the right, the artery is to the left, and the vein is most posterior.

Weigh and measure the liver, and record the appearance of its external surface. If the gallbladder is present, record its size as well. Begin the dissection at the liver hilum. Avoid the temptation to section the liver parenchyma before the hilar structures have been located, identified, and sampled. First, identify and submit a shave section of the common hepatic duct, the hepatic artery, and the portal vein. Next, take three transverse sections of the hilar structures and associated fat. Take one of these sections near the margin and the other two from the point where these structures branch into the right and left lobes of the liver. The aim is to obtain complete cross sections of the bile duct, hepatic artery, and portal vein for histologic evaluation. Look for lymph nodes in the hilar soft tissues, and sample each of these for histologic evaluation. Next, dissect the gallbladder from its bed, and process it as you would a routine cholecystectomy (see Chapter 14).

Now that the porta hepatis has been carefully examined and sampled, section the liver paren-

chyma. Using a long, sharp knife, section the liver as illustrated along its longest axis on either side of the hilum. This median section will show the maximum surface area of the cut liver parenchyma, and it will best demonstrate the branches of the hepatic ducts, hepatic arteries, and portal vein as they enter the liver. Serially section the detached portions of liver, cutting perpendicular to the original cut. Record the color and consistency of the liver parenchyma. Is the liver nodular, fibrotic, or necrotic? Are any focal lesions present?

In addition to the sections taken of the porta hepatis, all lobes of the liver should be represented in a routine sampling of the explanted liver. Three sections each from the right and left lobes, and one section each from the caudate and quadrate lobes are generally sufficient, but more sections may be required to sample all areas that have a distinct appearance. Additional sections should also be taken of any focal lesions.

Important Issues to Address in Your Surgical Pathology Report on Liver Explants

- What procedure was performed, and what structures/organs are present? How much does the liver weigh?
- What are the nature and extent of the disease that underlies the liver failure?
- Is the gallbladder present? Are calculi or any other pathologic processes identified?
- Is a neoplasm present? What are its type, grade, size, and location? Does the tumor involve the structures of the porta hepatis? Are the margins at the porta hepatis involved by tumor?
- How many lymph nodes were examined, and how many of them harbor a metastasis?

14 Gallbladder

Cholecystectomies

Gallbladders are one of the more frequently encountered specimens in the surgical pathology laboratory. They are usually removed for stones and/or inflammatory conditions, but rarely, they may harbor a neoplasm.

The gallbladder is a saccular structure with one end that narrows to form the cystic duct. Even though this structural anatomy is straightforward, take a moment to orient the specimen and identify a few important features. First, note that the gallbladder has two very different external surfaces. One side of the gallbladder is smooth and glistening, while the other is rough. The distinction between these two surfaces is important. The smooth surface is lined by peritoneum. In contrast, the rough surface is where the adventitia of the gallbladder has been dissected from the undersurface of the liver, and it represents a surgical margin. Second, the lymphatics of the gallbladder drain into a lymph node that is located along the cystic duct. When present in the specimen, this lymph node can be identified by palpating the soft tissues investing the cystic duct.

Measure the specimen, and describe the external surfaces. One important issue to address at the onset of the dissection is whether the specimen is received intact. Not uncommonly, a gallbladder will be opened in the operating room and the stones removed. Receipt of a previously opened gallbladder should be documented in the gross description. If the specimen is still intact, open the gallbladder lengthwise through its serosal-lined surface. Using a small pair of scissors, begin at the fundus, and extend the cut through the body and neck of the gallbladder and then through the cystic duct. The lumen of the cystic duct should be examined, even though the cystic duct may be tortuous and difficult to open. The direction in which the gallbladder is opened is not optional. Do not begin at the opening of the cystic duct, because a probe or scissors forced into this opening may dislodge stones.

After the specimen has been opened, note the contents of the gallbladder and the cystic duct. Specifically, look for calculi, and determine whether they are present within the lumen of the body of the gallbladder or within the cystic duct. Record the appearance of any calculi. Are they round or faceted? What is their color? Use a sharp blade to cut the calculi in half, and note the appearance of their cut surfaces. How many calculi are present? When numerous calculi are present, there is a tendency to give the size of the largest one. Instead, give the full range of sizes, keeping in mind that the smaller calculi are more apt to become lodged in the cystic duct than are the larger ones. Also note the thickness of the gallbladder wall, and describe the appearance of the mucosa. If a neoplasm is suggested by the presence of an exophytic or ulcerative lesion, then the external adventitial surface should be inked, as this represents a surgical margin.

The gallbladder is best sampled after it has been allowed to fix. For routine specimens, submit one representative full-thickness section from the fundus and one transverse section through the neck of the gallbladder. Additional sections are required when focal lesions are present. If a neoplastic process is suspected, ob-

Cholecystectomy

1. Orient the gallbladder. Distinguish the serosal surface from the adventitial surface. If present, locate the cystic duct lymph node.

2. Ink the adventitial surface margin if a tumor is suspected.

3. Open the gallbladder lengthwise through the serosal-lined portion. Begin at the fundus, and extend the incision through the cystic duct.

4. Record the number, size, and appearance of calculi. Note the location of any calculi, distinguishing between those in the gallbladder and those lodged in the cystic duct.

5. Submit representative sections from the fundus, the neck, and the cystic duct lymph node. Include additional sections of any focal lesions identified.

Open the gallbladder from the fundus toward the cystic duct.

Serosal surface

Adventitial surface

Sample the cystic duct lymph node.

Look for calculi lodged in the cystic duct.

Sample the neck and fundus for histology.

tain full-thickness sections of the tumor to demonstrate its maximum depth of invasion. Also submit sections from the periphery of the tumor to demonstrate its relationship to the surrounding uninvolved mucosa. To assess the status of the margins when a neoplasm is suspected, submit a shave section from the cystic duct margin and perpendicular sections from the inked adventitial surface. When present, the cystic duct lymph node should always be submitted for histologic evaluation.

Important Issues to Address in Your Surgical Pathology Report

- What procedure was performed, and what structures/organs are present?

- What are the nature and extent of the inflammatory processes (e.g., acute, chronic, xanthogranulomatous)? Be sure to mention the presence or absence of perforations and peritonitis.
- What are the contents of the gallbladder (e.g., bile, pus, blood, mucus)? When calculi are present, note their type (pigment, cholesterol, or mixed), number, and the range of sizes. Are any calculi lodged in the cystic duct?
- Is a neoplasm present? What are its type, grade, size, depth of invasion (mucosa, muscular layer, perimuscular connective tissue), and location? Does the tumor extend to the adventitial surface margin or to the cystic duct margin? Does the tumor extend into adjacent organs? Is this extension greater than 2 cm?
- How many lymph nodes were examined, and how many of them harbor a metastasis?

15 Pancreas

The pancreas can intimidate even the most experienced pathologist. The complexity of the anatomy of the pancreas and the importance of a good dissection in establishing the correct diagnosis make the arrival of a resected pancreas in the surgical pathology laboratory a particularly stressful event. This stress can, however, be greatly reduced if you familiarize yourself with a few basic aspects of the anatomy of the pancreas, and if you take a simple, logical approach to your dissection.

Pancreaticoduodenectomies

The Whipple procedure (pancreaticoduodenectomy) has emerged as an effective and safe treatment for neoplasms of the head of the pancreas, duodenum, distal common bile duct, and ampulla of Vater. The orientation of these specimens can be greatly simplified if you remember that the specimen is composed of four basic components: (1) the duodenum, (2) the ampulla of Vater, (3) the bile duct, and (4) the pancreas.

Begin by orienting the duodenum: two features of the duodenum can be used to identify its proximal and distal ends. First, the free proximal end is almost always shorter than the free distal segment of the resected duodenum. Second, a small part of the stomach is occasionally attached to the proximal end. Next, identify the bile duct. As illustrated, the common bile duct can be recognized by its greenish color and characteristic tubular appearance. Also, if the gallbladder is present, use the insertion of the cystic duct to identify the common bile duct. The remaining components of the pancreas can

be identified using the duodenum and bile duct as guides. The pancreas itself sits at the base of the junction of the bile duct and duodenum. The head of the pancreas sits within the duodenal C loop. The pancreatic neck margin can be recognized as the cut oval pancreatic surface with a central duct. Although the uncinate process of the pancreas is more difficult to identify, it can be visualized if you keep the anatomy of the pancreas in mind. As illustrated, the pancreas sits like a slightly curled hand enveloping the superior mesenteric artery and the portal vein. The thumb of the curled hand corresponds to the uncinate process of the pancreas and the flat fingers to the neck, body, and tail. Although the superior mesenteric vessels are not present in the resected specimen, remember that they were dissected from the pancreas right at the groove between the thumb and index finger.

After the major external landmarks have been identified, measure the dimensions of each, and ink the surface of the pancreas and the proximal and distal duodenal margins. Begin the dissection by opening the duodenum along the side opposite the pancreas. Look for and document any duodenal masses, ulcers, or areas of puckering of the duodenal mucosa. Before cutting the specimen any further, submit sections of the margins. These should include: (1) a shave section of the bile duct margin; (2) a shave section of the pancreatic neck margin; (3) a perpendicular section of the uncinate margin taken to include the vascular groove; (4) a perpendicular section from the proximal duodenal margin; and (5) a shave section from the distal duodenal margin. Next, using a pair of scissors, open the common bile duct. Because the extrapancreatic (proximal) portion of the duct is usually dilated, you may find it easier to start the incision at the proximal end. Extend the incision longitudinally down through the ampulla of Vater, and note any strictures or exophytic masses in the bile duct and in the ampulla of Vater. Similarly, if the gallbladder is present, open it from its dome through the cystic duct to the point where it opens into the common bile duct. Note any calculi, strictures, or masses, and take a representative section of the gallbladder for histology (see Chapter 14).

After the duodenum and bile duct have been opened, you can now section the pancreas. This can be accomplished in a variety of ways, but we like to bread-loaf it into 3-mm slices perpendicular to the long axis of the duodenum. Use a long sharp knife to cut through the pancreas, leaving each slice attached to the specimen at the duodenum.

Now that the various components of the specimen have been exposed, there are five questions to answer: First, is a neoplasm present? Most of the cancers will be obvious, but if you have trouble finding the tumor, look carefully at the bile duct. Often, the bile duct is strictured at the level of the tumor, and this stricture can be used to find the tumor. Second, if a tumor is present, where is it located, and what is its probable site of origin (pancreas, bile duct, ampulla of Vater, or duodenum)? Third, what is the size of the tumor (measured in centimeters)? Fourth, what is the gross appearance of the neoplasm (solid or cystic)? Finally, how many lymph nodes are present, and are the lymph nodes grossly abnormal? The answers to each of these five questions will help identify and stage the neoplasm, and each answer should be carefully documented in the gross description. At this point, fix the specimen overnight in formalin.

After the specimen has been well fixed, carefully paint the common bile duct with orange ink or tattoo powder. This simple step will help in the interpretation of microscopic slides, because without the paint in the bile duct, it can be almost impossible to distinguish the bile duct from the pancreatic duct microscopically. Next, submit sections for histology. The sections will flow naturally if you remember the four basic components of the specimen (the pancreas, duodenum, bile duct, and ampulla). Submit sections of the pancreatic parenchyma, the bile duct, the duodenum, the ampulla, and representative sections of all masses. Submit one section of pancreatic parenchyma for each 1 cm of maximum pancreatic length. As illustrated, a section that we find particularly helpful is a section parallel to the long axis of the bile duct that includes the duodenum, ampulla, bile duct, and pancreas all in one. If a mass is present, be sure to include sections that demonstrate the relationship of the mass to each of the four components of the specimen, and sections that demonstrate the relationship of the neoplasm to the anterior and posterior soft tissue margins. Next, submit a representative section of each lymph node. Although the lymphatic drainage of the pancreas is complex, we have not found detailed accounts of the exact location of each lymph node submitted to be helpful. Instead, we prefer to spend time making sure that we find all of the nodes. A good place to look for nodes is in the peripancreatic fat at the junction of the pancreas and duodenum. They may also be found in the mesentery and around the bile duct.

Distal Pancreatectomies

Distal pancreatectomies are much easier to handle than are pancreaticoduodenectomies. The anatomy is simple, and there are fewer margins to sample. First, find the proximal and distal ends of the pancreas. The spleen helps identify the distal aspect of the gland, and the cut surface of the pancreas is the proximal end. Next, weigh and measure the specimen, and submit a shave section of the proximal pancreatic margin. Ink the surface of the gland, and then bread-loaf it into 3-mm slices using a long sharp knife. These slices should be made perpendicular to the long axis of the gland. Examine the pancreatic parenchyma carefully, paying particular attention to the pancreatic duct. Is the duct dilated or stenotic? Are there any masses or calculi in it? What is the consistency of any fluid in the duct? Note the size, location, and gross appearance of any masses. Submit representative sections of any tumors and of the pancreatic parenchyma. Examine the peripancreatic soft tissues for lymph nodes, note their gross appearance, and submit a representative section of each. If the spleen is present, weigh it, measure it, section it,

Gallbladder

Surgical resection line

Bile duct

Neck

Body

Duodenum

Tail

Ampulla of Vater

Head of pancreas

Uncinate process

Superior mesenteric artery and portal vein

Use your left hand to simulate the anatomy of the pancreas.

Proximal duodenal margin

Bile duct margin

Pancreatic neck margin

Uncinate margin

Distal duodenal margin

Ampulla of Vater

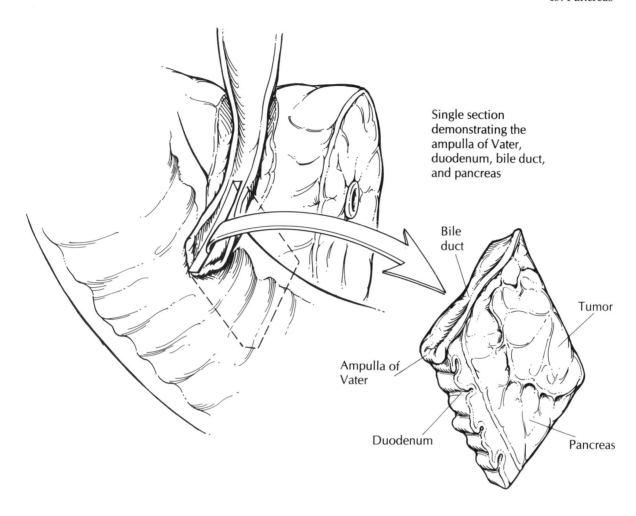

Single section
demonstrating the
ampulla of Vater,
duodenum, bile duct,
and pancreas

Bile
duct

Tumor

Ampulla of
Vater

Duodenum

Pancreas

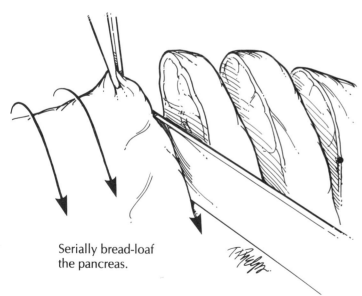

Serially bread-loaf
the pancreas.

Pancreaticoduodenectomy

1. Remember the four basic components of the specimen: the duodenum, the ampulla of Vater, the bile duct, and the pancreas.

2. Orient the specimen. The distal portion of the duodenum is usually longer than the proximal portion.

3. Shave the distal duodenal, bile duct, and pancreatic neck margins. Take perpendicular sections of the proximal duodenal and uncinate margins.

4. Open the duodenum on the side opposite the pancreas. Open the bile duct, and paint it with orange tattoo powder or orange ink.

5. Section the pancreas at 3-mm intervals.

6. Submit the five margin sections and sections of the tumor, the pancreatic parenchyma, the bile duct, the duodenum, the ampulla of Vater, and each lymph node.

and submit representative sections, as described in the discussion of the spleen (see Chapter 38).

Like the pancreaticoduodenectomy specimen, your final report should document the presence or absence of a neoplasm; the type, grade, and size of the tumor; the status of the margins; any lymph node metastases; and the presence or absence of vascular, perineural, and soft tissue invasion.

Cystic Tumors

Cystic masses in the pancreas should be handled as described above. In addition, remember to do the following: (1) Describe the character of the cyst contents. Is the fluid clear or cloudy? Is it serous, mucinous, or bloody? A good description of the cyst contents can be invaluable in determining the tumor type. (2) Document whether the cyst is unilocular or multilocular. How large are the cysts, and are there any mural nodules? (3) If the cyst is lined by mucinous epithelium, then the entire cyst should be submitted for histological diagnosis. Keep in mind that otherwise benign-appearing mucinous cystic neoplasms can harbor small invasive cancers.

Important Issues to Address in Your Surgical Pathology Report on Pancreatic Resections

- What procedure was performed, and what structures/organs are present?
- Is a neoplasm present?
- What is the probable site of origin of the tumor (bile duct, pancreas, ampulla of Vater, or duodenum)?
- What is the size of the tumor (in centimeters)?
- What are the histologic type and grade of the neoplasm? Is an *in situ* component identified?
- Does the tumor extend into the peripancreatic soft tissues? If so, does it extend anteriorly or posteriorly?
- Does the tumor infiltrate blood vessels, lymphatics, or nerves? Does the tumor extend into the pancreas, duodenum, ampulla of Vater, common bile duct, or spleen?
- Does the tumor involve any of the margins (pancreatic neck, uncinate, bile duct, soft tissue, and proximal and distal duodenal)?
- Does the tumor involve regional lymph nodes? Include the number of nodes examined and the number of nodes involved.
- Do the non-neoplastic portions of the pancreas and duodenum show any pathology?

IV   The Cardiovascular/ Respiratory System

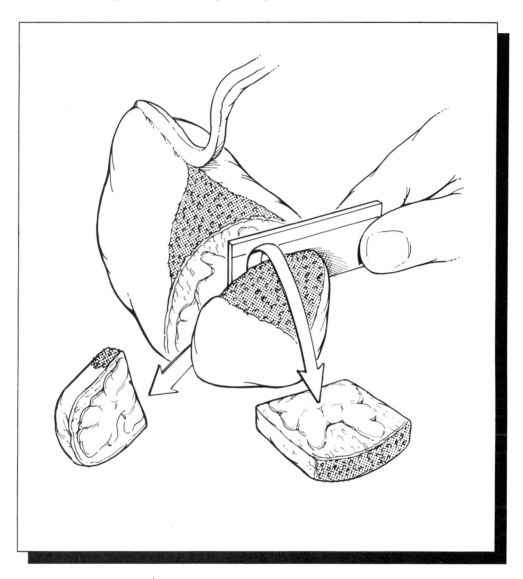

16 Heart Valves and Vessels

Heart Valves

For years, almost all valvular heart disease has been ascribed to chronic rheumatic heart disease. As a result, excised heart valves are frequently the most neglected specimens in the surgical pathology laboratory. Failure to pay appropriate attention to resected valves can be a disservice to the patient. Careful examination of heart valves not only will help in the clinical management of these patients, but may also help in the development of improved prosthetic heart valves.

As is true for any specimen, clinical information is essential for the appropriate classification of heart valve disease. The results of echocardiography and cardiac catheterization, as well as the surgeon's operative findings, should all be obtained before you begin your examination. Although there is some overlap, the examination of native, mechanical, and bioprosthetic heart valves each presents unique challenges.

Native Heart Valves

Although we tend to think of heart valves as consisting only of the valve leaflets, remember the other components of the valve. The atrioventricular valves (mitral and tricuspid) are composed of an annulus, leaflets, chordae tendineae, and papillary muscles. The semilunar valves (the aortic and pulmonic) are made up of three cusps, each with a sinus. These cusps meet at three commissures. Remembering these basic components of each valve is essential, because, although some native heart valves can be removed intact by the surgeon, the majority are fragmented during removal.

Before handling an excised valve, check to see if cultures need to be taken. In addition, a photograph of the inflow and outflow aspects of a valve can help document the cause of the disease. Similarly, a radiograph of the specimen may help establish the extent and distribution of calcifications. Begin by documenting whether the valve is in one piece or is fragmented. Note the dimensions of the valve as well as the dimensions of the valve orifice. Next, systematically examine each component of the valve. Start with the leaflets. Count and record the number of leaflets. Note the edges of the leaflets, and look for any evidence of rolling or commissural fusion. Next, examine the leaflets themselves. Document the presence or absence of myxoid changes, fibrosis, calcifications, thrombi, and vegetations. If the leaflets are fibrotic, are they diffusely or focally involved? If calcifications or thrombi are present, document their location, size, and apparent impact on valve function. If vegetations are noted, are they friable or firm? Next, for atrioventricular valves, examine the chordae tendineae and papillary muscles. Are the chordae normal, or are they shortened, thickened, stretched, fused, or ruptured? Are the papillary muscles normal, or is there evidence of recent or remote myocardial infarction? If a portion of the annulus is present, examine it as well. Once you have completed your gross description, submit a section for histology. The section should include the valve leaflet, the free edge of the valve, and if present, the chordae and papillary muscle. It may be necessary to decalcify this section.

Starr-Edwards
(Ball-in-cage mechanical)

St. Jude
(Bileaflet mechanical)

Bjork-Shiley
(Monoleaflet mechanical)

Medtronic-Hall
(Monoleaflet mechanical)

Carpentier-Edwards and
Hancock porcine
(Tissue valves)

Common Prosthetic Cardiac Valves

1. Identify the type of valve.

2. Look for, document the presence of, and sample for histology any thrombi, vegetations, or fibrous tissue proliferations.

3. Document the movement of the valve.

4. Examine and document the condition of each component of the valve: (1) the valve ring, (2) the occluder or poppet, and (3) components that limit the movement of the poppet or allow the occluder to tilt.

5. *Save the valve. It's the law.*

Mechanical Heart Valves

Numerous different types of mechanical heart valves have been developed over the years. The majority of these valves have three main components (1) a cloth ring, which is used by the surgeon to sew the valve in place; (2) an occluder or poppet (ball or disk); and (3) components that limit the movement of the poppet or allow the occluder to tilt. Despite the similarities, the various types of mechanical heart valves have several important differences, and different valves are prone to different complications. Therefore, before beginning your examination of a mechanical heart valve, we recommend that you identify the type of valve by referring to a valve identification book such as "Cardiac Valve Identification Atlas and Guide," in *Guide to Prosthetic Cardiac Valves*.[2] Examples of some of the more common types of mechanical and bioprosthetic valves are illustrated here.

Next, the valve can be cultured, photographed, and x-rayed as indicated. Try out the movement of the valve. Does the valve apparatus open and close fully? Thrombi can form at the junction of the various components of the valve, especially at cloth-metal interfaces. These thrombi are important to identify, because they can be a source of emboli or a nidus for the development of an infection, and they may interfere with valve function. Document the location and size of any thrombi or vegetations, and note whether or not they interfere with valve function. Some valves incite an intense overgrowth of fibrous tissue, and this fibrous tissue can cause valve dysfunction and even luminal stenosis. Therefore, it is important to note the presence or absence of fibrous tissue. Finally, carefully look for evidence of wear and tear on the various mechanical components of the valve. Is there any evidence of cracking or disk wear? As is true for natural heart valves, the effect of any pathology on valve function should be carefully documented. In most cases, it is not possible to submit any tissue for histologic examination, but if vegetations are present, a section should be submitted for histology. Remember that if you discover that harm or death has come to a patient because of a malfunctioning prosthetic heart valve, in the United States, the U.S. Safe Medical Devices Act of 1990 (Public Law 101-629) requires you to notify either the manufacturer or the Food and Drug Administration. Finally, as is true for all mechanical devices removed surgically, be sure to save the valve, because it may need to be returned to the manufacturer.

Bioprosthetic Heart Valves

A variety of bioprosthetic heart valves are used. These include (1) porcine aortic valves, (2) bovine and pericardial valves, and (3) human aortic homographs. As is true for the native and mechanical heart valves, the first step should be to ask yourself if the valve needs to be cultured, photographed, or x-rayed. Next, carefully inspect the valve leaflets for thrombi, vegetations, calcifications, and evidence of fibrous overgrowth. In particular, look for evidence of tears or perforations in the valve leaflets. Again, make sure to document both the location and size of any lesions and to describe the effect of these lesions on valve function. If a sewing ring is present, be sure to examine it as well.

Important Issues to Address in Your Surgical Pathology Report on Heart Valves

Native Heart Valves

- How many leaflets are present?
- Do the leaflets show evidence of fusion, myxoid change, fibrosis, calcification, thrombi, or vegetations?
- Do the chordae show evidence of shortening, thickening, stretching, fusion, or rupture?
- Are the papillary muscles infarcted?
- Do any of these changes appear to have an impact on valve function?

Mechanical and Bioprosthetic Valves

- What type of valve is it?
- Is there evidence of thrombi, fibrous tissue overgrowth, wear and tear, or mechanical failure?
- Is the valve function compromised?

Arteries and Veins

The examination of arteries and veins is straightforward, particularly if one remembers the three layers of each: the intima, media, and adventitia. Measure the length and external and internal diameters of the vessel. Examine the lumen for thrombi, examine the intima for evidence of intimal proliferations such as atherosclerosis, and document the percentage of luminal narrowing caused by any lesions. Examine the media for evidence of aneurysm formation or fibromuscular hyperplasia. Take sections that are both longitudinal and perpendicular to the long axis of the vessel. The longitudinal sections will be particularly helpful in demonstrating alterations involving the media, and the perpendicular sections can demonstrate the effect of any lesion on the luminal diameter.

Temporal Artery Biopsies

Biopsies are occasionally taken of the temporal artery in cases for which temporal arteritis is suspected. These biopsies need to be carefully and thoroughly examined, at multiple levels, for focal disease. The average biopsy is about 12 mm long. Cut it into four pieces, each about 3 mm long, and have the laboratory embed each piece on end. We like to get four sets of step sections through the block, each set containing three hematoxylin and eosin stained sections, one elastin stained (Verhoeff's/van Gieson's), and one unstained. Thus, one temporal artery biopsy produces at least 16 slides to examine.

17 Lungs

General Comments

Pathologists are routinely called on to process a diverse spectrum of lung specimens, ranging in size and complexity from minute biopsies to pneumonectomies. Despite this diversity, these specimens can be systematically approached by keeping in mind the five basic components of the lung specimen: the airways, the lung parenchyma, the pleura, the vessels, and the lymph nodes.

Before beginning the dissection, be sure to ask yourself two questions: First, does the pathology need to be revealed immediately? For example, if an infection is suspected, cultures may have to be taken from fresh tissues in a sterile fashion. Likewise, in the case of a suspected neoplasm, frozen section evaluation may be required to establish a diagnosis or to assess resection margins, and sampling of fresh tissue may be needed for ancillary diagnostic studies, such as electron microscopy. Next, ask which method of dissection will most effectively reveal the pathologic process and best demonstrate the relationship of the disease to the surrounding lung and pleura. There is more than one way to dissect a lung, and the method of sectioning is often dictated by the type of specimen, the suspected nature of the pathologic process, and the size and location of the pathologic process. Clearly, the more clinical information that is available, including radiographic findings, the more effectively these questions can be answered. Finally, keep in mind that a wealth of information can be obtained simply by palpating the intact specimen. Even small focal lesions can be appreciated by palpation, and this fast and easy method of examination should become a routine part of the initial evaluation of any lung resection.

Limited Pulmonary Resections

Limited pulmonary resections include open lung biopsies and wedge resections for both neoplastic and non-neoplastic diseases. These specimens are generally taken from the periphery of the lung. As illustrated, they usually are wedge-shaped pieces of lung tissue invested by visceral pleura. Because of their small size and peripheral location, lymph nodes and major bronchi are usually not present. Surgical staple lines may be present, and these represent the parenchymal resection margins. Document the dimensions of the specimen and the appearance of the pleural surface. If clinically indicated, fresh tissue can be harvested for microbial cultures and for immunofluorescence. If immediate dissection is not required, however, fix the specimen before proceeding with the dissection. Fixation in distention can be accomplished by gently infusing formalin directly into the lung parenchyma at several sites through a small-gauge needle. Take care not to overdistend the specimen. Submerge the distended specimen in formalin until it is well fixed. Following fixation, trim the staple lines from the specimen. Be careful not to remove too much lung tissue with these staples, because the exposed lung parenchyma immediately adjacent to the staples represents a surgical margin. Dry and ink the exposed parenchymal margin, and then serially section the specimen in a plane perpen-

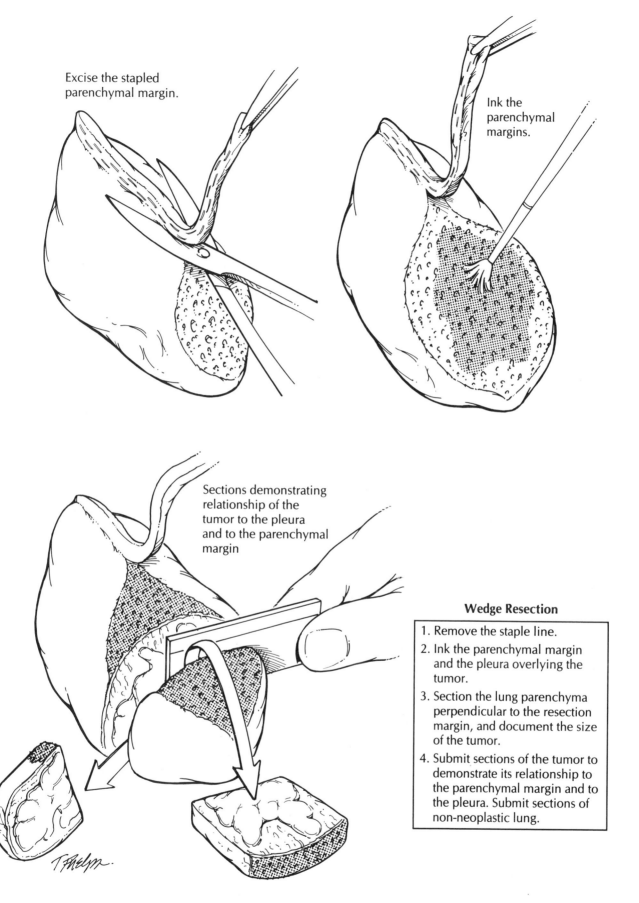

Excise the stapled parenchymal margin.

Ink the parenchymal margins.

Sections demonstrating relationship of the tumor to the pleura and to the parenchymal margin

T.Phelan.

Wedge Resection

1. Remove the staple line.
2. Ink the parenchymal margin and the pleura overlying the tumor.
3. Section the lung parenchyma perpendicular to the resection margin, and document the size of the tumor.
4. Submit sections of the tumor to demonstrate its relationship to the parenchymal margin and to the pleura. Submit sections of non-neoplastic lung.

83

dicular to that of the parenchymal resection margin.

After sectioning the specimen, evaluate the lung for focal and diffuse processes, and describe these findings. For neoplasms, note the size of the tumor, the appearance of its cut surface, and the relationship of the tumor to the pleura and to the surrounding lung parenchyma. Note also the distance from the edge of the tumor to the resection margin. Submit one to four sections of the lesion (depending on its size), selecting sections that demonstrate the tumor's relationship to the pleura, to adjacent lung tissue, and to the parenchymal resection margin. Sample the parenchymal margin, using perpendicular sections when the tumor closely approaches the margin. In addition, submit two sections of non-neoplastic lung. Intrapulmonary lymph nodes and bronchi will generally not be present in these peripheral lung biopsies, but if they are present, they should be sampled.

For non-neoplastic lung diseases, submit the vast majority of the specimen for histologic evaluation. In selected instances, some material should be fresh-frozen, especially if immunofluorescence studies are needed to establish a diagnosis. Note the size of the airspaces, the patency of any airways that are present, and the crepitance of the parenchyma. Only rarely should intraoperative frozen section consultations be performed for non-neoplastic lung disease.

Lobectomies and Pneumonectomies

The largest lung specimens consist of lobectomies and pneumonectomies. These procedures are usually done to remove neoplasms. When a tumor directly invades beyond the pleura, these specimens may also include an en bloc resection of the involved adjacent structures (e.g., chest wall, left atrium, or diaphragm).

Weigh, measure, and anatomically orient the specimen while it is fresh. One quick and easy way to orient the specimen is to inspect the structures at the lung hilum. On the left side, the pulmonary artery is situated superior to the airway, while on the right side, it is situated anterior to the airway. Also, the right side has three lobes; whereas the left side has two and a prominent lingular segment. Carefully inspect the pleural surfaces. Look for the presence of pleural retraction, because this finding suggests the presence of an underlying neoplasm. Palpate the intact specimen: Is the tumor located centrally or peripherally? Which lobe of the lung appears to be involved? Does the tumor extend across a fissure to involve more than one lobe? Apply ink to the pleura overlying the tumor.

If immediate dissection of the specimen is not required, it is best to fix the specimen in distention. Infuse formalin directly into the large airways, and submerge the entire specimen in formalin for overnight fixation. Take care not to overdistend the lung.

If you remember each of the five basic components of the lung (airways, lymph nodes, vessels, parenchyma, and pleura), then your description and dissection can be carried out in a simple and systematic fashion. Many proximal lung tumors arise from the airways, and so we find it most helpful to start the dissection with the airways. Begin by removing the bronchial and vascular margins as shave sections. Next, expose the bronchial mucosa by opening the large airways out to the subsegmental branches with small scissors. Carefully examine the mucosa of the airways, because subtle changes in the appearance of the mucosa may indicate a premalignant lesion. Similarly, open the large pulmonary vessels and evaluate them for invasion by tumor.

By dissecting the larger airways, you have opportunely exposed the regional lymph nodes, and these should be sampled at this time. Direct the search for lymph nodes to the soft tissues at the hilum and to the lung parenchyma immediately surrounding the airways. Lymph nodes are often easily visualized by their black (anthracotic) pigmentation. It is generally not necessary to further designate these lymph nodes. Although the status of the various mediastinal lymph node groups is crucial to the staging of lung tumors, these groups are not routinely part of the lobectomy/pneumonectomy specimen. Rather, they are usually separately submitted and labeled by the surgeon.

Section the lung parenchyma in the plane that best reveals the pathologic process and its relationship to the surrounding structures of the lung. For proximal lung tumors, this relationship can best be demonstrated by sectioning the lung along the plane of the involved airways. As illustrated, this can be accomplished by first placing probes into the airways that have already been partially opened and then using these probes to help guide your knife through the lung parenchyma. In this manner, one can determine the origin and size of proximal tumors and evaluate the lung parenchyma distal to the tumor. The remaining lung parenchyma can then be sectioned at 1-cm intervals. For peripherally located tumors, a site of origin from an airway may not be apparent. In these instances, serial sections through the tumor perpendicular to the closest segmental bronchus may best reveal the relationships of the tumor to the pleura, to the surrounding lung parenchyma, and to the small airways.

For non-neoplastic lung diseases, section the specimen in a manner that best correlates with the radiographic studies. For example, thin serial sections of the fixed specimen in the transverse plane can be used to arrive at a one-to-one correlation between changes identified in computed tomography scans and the pathology. In the description of these large lung specimens, do not lose sight of the systematic approach that includes descriptions of all five basic components of the lung.

For specimens that harbor a neoplasm, the major aims of tissue sampling for histology are to document the tumor type, the origin of the tumor, the extent of the tumor (local and metastatic), and the adequacy of tumor resection. To assess tumor type, submit four sections of tumor, both from the center of the tumor and from the interface of the tumor with the surrounding lung tissue. Make every effort to demonstrate the relationship of the tumor to an associated airway. For more proximal tumors with an apparent endobronchial component, take sections along the involved airway to include both tumor and bronchus. For peripheral lesions, a site of origin from a small airway may not be apparent. In these cases, take sections through the tumor in a plane perpendicular to the airways. Document tumor extension to or

through the pleura with sections taken at right angles to the pleura in areas of retraction. Similarly, take sections of tumor extension into the pulmonary vessels, hilar soft tissues, and chest wall. Submit representative sections of all lymph nodes identified in the hilar and peribronchial regions. If the specimen also contains a portion of chest wall, take sections and margins from all of the attached structures (parietal pleura, skin, soft tissues, and ribs), as if this block were its own specimen. Finally, submit sections of non-neoplastic lung from each lobe, including sections taken distal to the tumor for documentation of an obstructive pneumonic process.

For diffuse non-neoplastic processes, submit representative sections of lung parenchyma from each lobe as well as sections of proximal airways. If a focal lesion is encountered, section it in the manner described above for a neoplasm.

Important Issues to Address in Your Surgical Pathology Report on Lung Resections

- What procedure was performed, and what structures/organs are present?
- Is a neoplasm present?
- How large is the tumor, and where is it located?
- What are the histologic type and grade of the tumor?
- Does the tumor infiltrate the large airways, pleura, or vessels?
- What is the status of each of the margins (parenchymal, pleural, vascular, and bronchial)?
- Is there any evidence of metastatic disease? Record the number of lymph nodes examined and the number of lymph node metastases.
- Is there any pathology in the non-neoplastic lung?

Shave the bronchial and
vascular margins.

Open the
airway.

Use probes in the airway to
guide the knife.

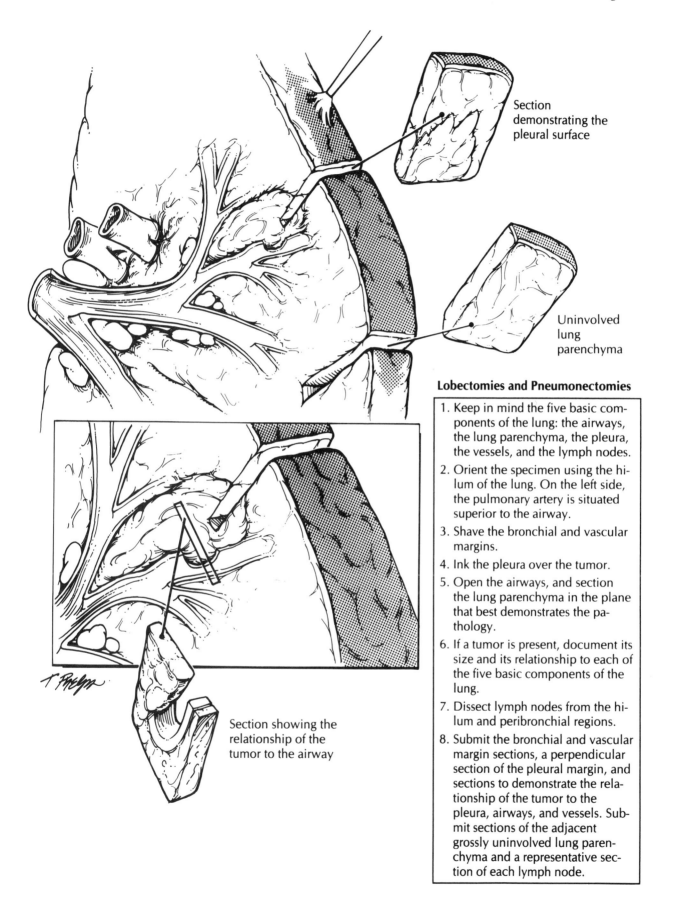

Section demonstrating the pleural surface

Uninvolved lung parenchyma

Section showing the relationship of tumor to the airway

Lobectomies and Pneumonectomies

1. Keep in mind the five basic components of the lung: the airways, the lung parenchyma, the pleura, the vessels, and the lymph nodes.

2. Orient the specimen using the hilum of the lung. On the left side, the pulmonary artery is situated superior to the airway.

3. Shave the bronchial and vascular margins.

4. Ink the pleura over the tumor.

5. Open the airways, and section the lung parenchyma in the plane that best demonstrates the pathology.

6. If a tumor is present, document its size and its relationship to each of the five basic components of the lung.

7. Dissect lymph nodes from the hilum and peribronchial regions.

8. Submit the bronchial and vascular margin sections, a perpendicular section of the pleural margin, and sections to demonstrate the relationship of the tumor to the pleura, airways, and vessels. Submit sections of the adjacent grossly uninvolved lung parenchyma and a representative section of each lymph node.

Bone, Soft Tissue, and Skin

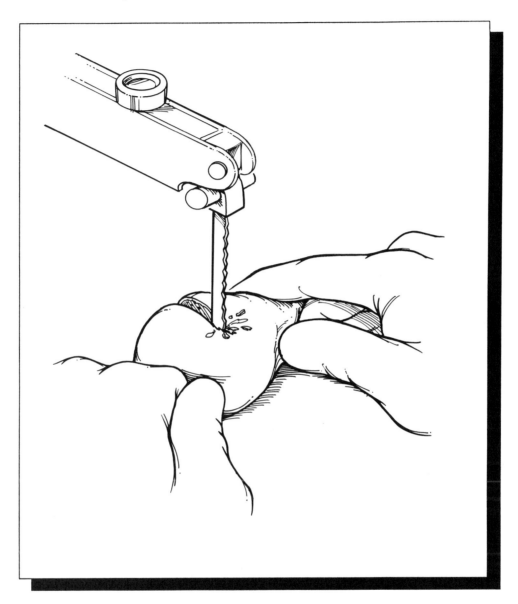

18 Bone

Edward F. McCarthy, Jr., M.D.

General Comments

The hardness of bone introduces three challenges that are unique to the dissection of bone specimens: (1) Many lesions involving bone are not easily appreciated simply by palpating and inspecting the intact specimen. This inability to pinpoint the lesion may frustrate attempts to demonstrate its size and location when cutting the bone specimen. (2) Bone specimens cannot be easily dissected and sampled with standard knives and scalpels. (3) Since the microtome blade also cannot penetrate bone, bone cannot easily be sectioned in the histology laboratory. Fortunately, each of these obstacles can be overcome. Specimen radiographs (Table 18-1) allow one to visualize the extent and location of the pathologic process so that the specimen can be cut in the proper plane; appropriate saws (Table 18-2) allow one to cut bone without destroying the specimen; and finally, special solutions (Table 18-3) can demineralize bone making it easier to section for microscopic evaluation. Thus, the successful dissection of bone speci-

mens requires that the prosector master the use of radiography, special techniques, instruments, and a variety of chemical solutions.

Small Bone Fragments

Whether dealing with bone biopsies, currettings, or the removal of small bones, there is always the danger of overdecalcifying the tissue. Efforts to minimize the time in decalcification solution and to separate out tissue fragments that do not require decalcification will reap great rewards when evaluating these tissues microscopically. When it is necessary to cut a bone fragment before processing, orient and cut the bone to show as much surface as possible. For example, small tubular bones such as metatarsals or ribs should be cut longitudinally rather than in cross section. When articular cartilage is present, sections should be taken to show its relationship to cortical bone. For specimens consisting of multiple pieces of tissue, soft tissues should be separated from bone and processed routinely in formalin without decalcification, while pieces of bone should be grouped in cassettes according to size and density to allow for uniform decalcification.

Large Bone Specimens

Femoral heads are the most common example of large bone specimens. They are usually removed because of either osteoarthritis or a hip fracture. Consequently, it is particularly important to identify, inspect, and sample the articu-

---

TABLE 18-1. X-raying specimens.

- An ideal x-ray source is the Faxitron machine—an x-ray machine that is small enough to be kept in the surgical pathology cutting area.

- Take two radiographs of the specimen: one to show the antero-posterior view and the other to show the lateral view.

- Using the findings of the radiograph, cut the specimen in the plane that best demonstrates the lesion. For example, if the lesion is best seen in the antero-posterior view, then cut the specimen in the coronal plane.

TABLE 18-2. Cutting specimens.

- Choose the right saw:

Vibrating table saw	Band saw
Minimizes artifact that is due to bone dust or crushing of the tissue.	Creates bone crush and bone dust artifact.
Relatively safe.	**Dangerous!** (Keep your hands away from the blade.) Have an assistant help hold and guide the specimen.
Inadequate for very large specimens or very dense bone.	Cuts large specimens and dense bone with ease.

- Do not use the band saw to cut through soft tissues (unless the soft tissues are frozen solid).

- Cut the bone longitudinally in the plane that shows the maximum area of diseased bone.

- When serially sectioning bone, the bone slices should be of uniform thickness, not to exceed 3–4 mm.

- Remove bone dust from the cut surfaces of the specimen. Gentle rinsing with saline or water and brushing with a soft toothbrush works quite well.

lar surface and any fracture site. Measure the specimen and describe the articular cartilage, noting whether it is eroded, frayed, pitted, or absent. The presence of osteophytes should also be noted. As illustrated, separate the dome of the femoral head from the neck, then place the cut surface of the head on the table saw, and section it into 3-mm slices in a plane perpendicular to the articular cartilage. Note the density of the bone and the thickness of the cartilage. In a similar manner, serially section the femoral neck. Look for the presence of blood clot, marrow hemorrhage, or a neoplasm.

Sampling for histology should be guided by the clinical history and gross findings. For cases of osteoarthritis, sample the femoral head to show cartilage destruction and the reaction of the underlying bone. In cases of fracture, direct your attention to the fracture site; most of the sections should come from this area. Always submit at least one cassette of soft tissue including the synovial membrane and capsule.

TABLE 18-3. Decalcifying specimens.

- Fix tissues in formalin before decalcifying.

- Decalcification obscures cellular detail:
    Never decalcify a specimen over the weekend. Specimen decalcification should be monitored daily.
    If the tissue permits, submit at least one section of tumor without decalcification. This section may be more suitable for histologic evaluation and immunohistochemical analysis.

- Thin sections of uniform thickness permit a faster and more even decalcification process.

Segmental Resections and Amputations for Neoplasms

Segmental Resections

Segmental resections of bone are performed for malignant neoplasms and aggressive benign tumors. Because local recurrence is an important complication, the margins of resection need to be carefully evaluated. The soft tissue margins are best sampled while the specimen is intact and still easy to orient. After inking the soft tissue resection margin, sample the margin using perpendicular sections from those areas for which there is gross or radiologic suspicion of margin involvement (see Chapter 6 for a description of sampling margins from a complex specimen).

After soft tissue margins are sampled, decide which plane of section will best demonstrate the lesion. The radiographic findings will help guide this strategy. For the saw to cleanly pass through the bone, expose the surfaces of the bone as illustrated by cutting through and peeling back the soft tissues in this plane. Next, bisect the bone in the appropriate plane (usually the coronal plane) using a band saw. Inspect the cut surface. The extent of the lesion should then be measured and described. In addition, the presence of cortical penetration and soft tissue extension should be noted. Look for noncontiguous "skip" lesions in the medullary canal, and measure the distance from the edges of the tumor to the bone resection margin. Scoop a

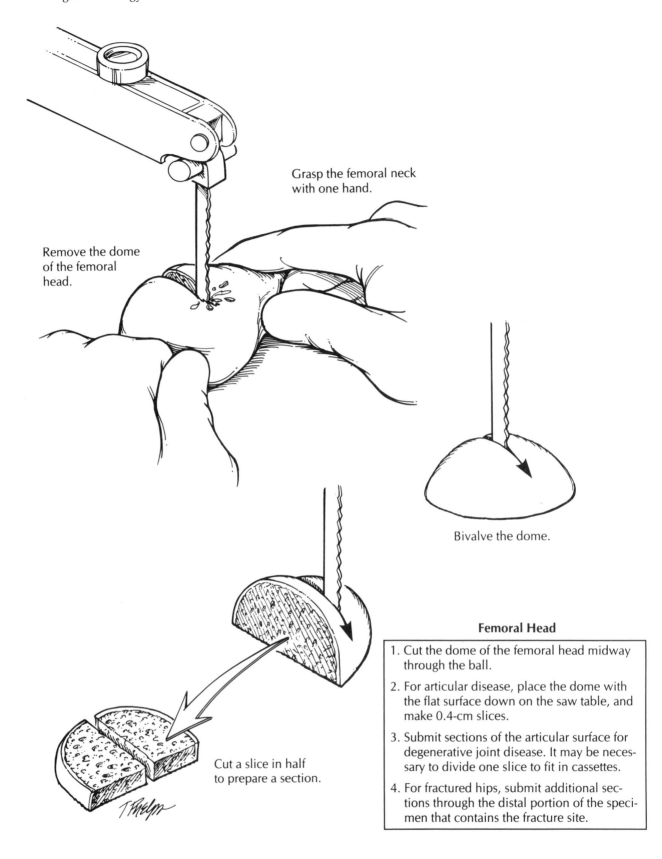

Remove the dome of the femoral head.

Grasp the femoral neck with one hand.

Bivalve the dome.

Cut a slice in half to prepare a section.

Femoral Head

1. Cut the dome of the femoral head midway through the ball.

2. For articular disease, place the dome with the flat surface down on the saw table, and make 0.4-cm slices.

3. Submit sections of the articular surface for degenerative joint disease. It may be necessary to divide one slice to fit in cassettes.

4. For fractured hips, submit additional sections through the distal portion of the specimen that contains the fracture site.

Remove the soft tissue overlying the bone.

Bivalve the specimen.

Make a parallel cut to produce a 0.4-cm thick slab.

Make sections to match a grid on the photocopy.

Bone Tumors

1. When the bone lesion has little or no soft tissue involvement, dissect the soft tissue off the bone.

2. Orient the segment of bone so that the saw produces a cut surface to show the lesion that matches the radiographic image.

3. Make a parallel cut to produce a 0.4-cm slab.

4. Photocopy the slab. Make a grid on the copy, and section the slab to match the grid.

5. Submit sections of the soft tissue margins, bone margins, and if the patient was given preoperative therapy, the entire slab of the bone.

small amount of marrow from the end(s) of the bone, and submit this marrow as the bone margin(s).

An alternative method is to freeze the entire specimen. The frozen specimen does not require removal of the soft tissues before cutting the bone. Thus, the relationship of the bone neoplasm to soft tissue spread is better preserved.

Now you are ready to cut a slab from the face of the bone cut surface. Place one half of the bisected specimen on the band saw, and cut a complete 4-mm-thick slab, then photograph and x-ray the slab. Ideally, this slab should be thin, uniform, and represent the greatest surface area of the tumor. Before sectioning the slab further, make a representation of the slab to map the precise location of each section submitted for histology. One method is to photocopy the slab and then to draw grids slightly smaller than your cassette size on the photocopy. The entire slab can then be blocked out and submitted for microscopic examination according to the grids on the photocopy.

When the patient has received neoadjuvant chemotherapy, the entire face of the slab should be evaluated microscopically to determine the percentage of tumor necrosis. When the patient has not received neoadjuvant chemotherapy, you may be more selective in the sections that you submit for histology. Important areas that should always be sampled include: (1) the intramedullary component of the neoplasm; (2) penetration of the tumor through the cortex; (3) extension of the tumor into soft tissues; (4) the interface of the tumor with normal bone; (5) involvement by the tumor of an articular surface and/or joint space; and (6) the bone margin(s).

Amputation Specimens

Although amputations for tumor appear more complex than segmental resections as a result of their size and bulk, they can be dissected along the same guidelines given for segmental resections. Indeed, after margins are sampled, the portion of the limb containing the bones and joints not involved by the neoplasm can be removed. This, in essence, converts the specimen to one that is similar to the segmental resection.

The dissection of amputations performed because of gangrene is described in Chapter 41.

Important Issues to Address in Your Surgical Pathology Report on Bone Tumors

- What procedure was performed, and what structures/organs are present?
- What type of neoplasm is present?
- What are the size and histologic grade of the neoplasm?
- If the patient received neoadjuvant chemotherapy, what is the percentage of tumor necrosis?
- Is there any cortical penetration or soft tissue invasion?
- What is the status of the soft tissue and bone margins of resection?
- Is a skip lesion present?

19 Soft Tissue, Nerves, and Muscle

Soft Tissue

Soft tissue resections are often complex specimens containing soft tissues, skin, and sometimes even bone. The general approach to these specimens is a simple one, and it parallels that outlined for complex head and neck specimens in Chapter 6. First, identify the various components of the specimen (soft tissue, bone, and skin). Second, think of each component as a geometric shape. Third, approach each component separately. Fourth, look for relationships between any lesions and each component.

With the general approach outlined above in mind, start the dissection by orienting the specimen. Do not hesitate to ask the surgeon to help with this step. Large muscle bundles move easily relative to one another. A margin that looks close in fact may have been covered by a large bundle of muscle that has shifted. The only way to be sure that tissue has not shifted is to discuss the specimen with the surgeon. Next, make sure that you know the anatomy. The origin of a sarcoma from a nerve can be missed if one is not familiar with the anatomic location of the major nerves in the specimen. After the specimen has been oriented and the anatomy determined, identify the various components of the specimen (soft tissue, bone, skin, etc.). This step helps ensure that important components of the specimen are not left out of the dissection.

Next, measure the overall dimensions of the specimen, and document the size of each individual component. The external appearance of each component can then be described. In particular, note the size and position of any biopsy sites.

The next step is to sample the margins. The evaluation of the margins of a large complex specimen is simplified by thinking of each component of the specimen as a geometric shape. As illustrated in Chapter 6, the soft tissue can usually be thought of as a cube, the bone as a cylinder and, if present, the skin as a square sheet. Ink the specimen, and take sections to demonstrate the margins of each of the components. There are usually six soft tissue margins (a cube has six sides), and these can be taken as perpendicular margins. These margins usually include the anterior, posterior, medial, lateral, inferior, and superior surfaces. Similarly, there are usually four skin margins (a square has four sides), and these can be taken as perpendicular margins. Shave sections of the bone (the ends of a cylinder), vascular, and neural margins should also be taken.

The specimen can now be sectioned. Determine the location and long axis of the tumor by palpating the specimen and reviewing the preoperative computed tomography (CT) scans. Section the specimen using a long sharp knife in the plane that will demonstrate the largest cross section of the tumor. Carefully document the size, consistency, and color of the tumor. Measure twice, because size is one of the most important predictors of outcome for patients with a soft tissue tumor. Also note any cysts and areas of necrosis, hemorrhage, calcification, myxoid change, bone formation, or cartilage, and whether or not the edge of the tumor is encapsulated, pushing, or infiltrative. It may be helpful to correlate the gross appearance of the

Soft Tissue Tumor Resections

1. Orient the specimen. This step frequently requires close cooperation between the surgeon and the pathologist.

2. Be familiar with the regional anatomy.

3. Ink the soft tissue and skin margins of the specimen.

4. Think of each component of the specimen (i.e., bone, soft tissue, and skin) as a geometric shape, and take perpendicular or shave margins of each component.

5. Section the specimen to demonstrate the long axis of the tumor.

6. Submit portions of tumor for possible electron microscopy and cytogenetics. Submit sections to demonstrate the relationship of the tumor to each of the components of the specimen. Include one section of tumor for every 1 cm of tumor diameter. Submit the indicated margin sections and any lymph nodes.

tumor with radiographic findings. For example, if calcifications are seen in a particular area of the tumor on CT scan, then that area should be identified grossly.

Next, document the distance of the tumor to each of the margins and the relationship of the tumor to each of the various components of the specimen. Is the tumor centered on or does it extend into the skin, muscle, periosteum, bone, joint, major vessels, or major nerves? This component of the dictation is important because it not only will help stage the tumor, but it can also help identify the site of origin of the tumor. Document the number of lymph nodes present, and sample each for histology.

Finally, the tumor itself can be sampled. First, submit a representative piece in glutaraldehyde for possible electron microscopy. Next, as clinically indicated, submit fresh tissue for cytogenetics or other special studies. These studies may be particularly important in the pediatric patient (see Chapter 35). Finally, submit sections for routine histology. These should include sections that demonstrate the relationship of the tumor to each component of the specimen, sections that demonstrate the relationship of the tumor to the closest margins, and sections from any foci within the tumor that look different from other areas of the tumor. A useful rule of thumb is that one section should be submitted for every 1 cm of the maximum diameter of the tumor. As you take these sections, keep in mind that important indications of tumor grade

(cellularity, necrosis, mitoses, etc.) and differentiation may be present only focally in large masses.

Important Issues to Address in Your Surgical Pathology Report on Soft Tissue Tumors

- What procedure was performed, and what structures/organs are present?
- What are the size, type, and histologic grade of the neoplasm?
- Does the neoplasm extend into skin, muscle, periosteum, bone, a joint space, major vessels, or major nerves?
- Are any margins involved?
- Is there evidence of metastatic disease? Record the number of lymph nodes examined and the presence or absence of lymph node metastases.

Nerve and Muscle Biopsies

Nerve and muscle biopsies are subject to a variety of artifacts if they are not properly handled. Furthermore, the interpretation of nerve and muscle pathology frequently requires special studies, including electron microscopy and histochemistry. For these reasons, nerve and muscle biopsies are best handled directly by specialized laboratories. Each laboratory usually has its own protocol for handling these biopsies. A detailed discussion of these specimens is, therefore, beyond the scope of this book. However, you should be aware of a few basics in processing these specimens, in case you do not have access to a specialized neuromuscular laboratory when the biopsy is done.

Muscle biopsies are usually obtained as two strips of muscle approximately 3 × 0.5 cm, taken parallel to the direction of the muscle fibers. A portion of tissue should be stretched to its normal *in situ* length, pinned to a card, and placed immediately (in the operating room) in 4% buffered glutaraldehyde. Do *not* mince this piece for electron microscopy. The remainder of the biopsy should be transported in saline-moistened gauze (do not soak) to the pathology laboratory. A portion of the biopsy should then be immediately fresh-frozen, and the remainder fixed in formalin. To ensure that the fiber size in the biopsy reflects the *in situ* diameter, and to reduce artifacts caused by the extreme contractility of the tissue, this piece of muscle should also be stretched to its normal *in situ* length in the direction of the fibers. This can be accomplished with a special muscle clamp or simply by pinning the stretched biopsy to a stiff index card. Be careful not to overstretch the tissue, as this can cause artifacts as well. Muscle biopsies frozen in liquid nitrogen tend to develop ice crystal artifacts, so it is best to freeze the tissue in 2-methyl-butane (isopentane) cooled to dry ice temperature or below. When submitting muscle biopsies in formalin for histology, remember to submit both longitudinal and cross sections.

Diagnostic nerve biopsies to determine the cause of a neuropathy are usually obtained as 3- to 5-cm-long strips of the sural nerve. As was true for muscle biopsies, these should be processed immediately by a specialized neuromuscular laboratory. You should handle these biopsies only when they cannot be handled by a specialized laboratory. Do not stretch these biopsies! Instead, the biopsy is usually cut into four pieces. One piece should be submitted in 4% glutaraldehyde for electron microscopy, one submitted in formalin for routine microscopy, another fresh-frozen and stored at −70°C, and the fourth saved fresh in saline-moistened gauze for the neuromuscular laboratory. If you have to cut a nerve, be careful not to squash it while cutting. Pressure on the nerve can induce the artifactual appearance of demyelinization. As was true for muscle biopsies, the sections submitted for histology should include both longitudinal and cross sections.

If a nerve biopsy is performed simply to document the transection of a nerve, the specimen should be entirely submitted in formalin for routine paraffin embedding and sectioning.

20 Skin

Thomas D. Horn, M.D.

General Comments

Skin biopsies comprise a large component of the volume of many anatomic pathology laboratories. These biopsies come in many shapes and sizes, both because of the ease with which the cutaneous surface can be sampled and also because biopsies are performed using a wide variety of techniques. Specimens are generally obtained to diagnose tumors, to ensure complete excision of tumors, and to identify or confirm the nature of cutaneous inflammatory diseases. Understanding the suspected diagnosis and purpose of the procedure will help expedite the processing of the tissue and ensure an accurate diagnosis.

Small Biopsies

Specimens obtained to establish the diagnosis of a cutaneous tumor are usually performed by the shave biopsy technique, punch biopsy technique, or curettage. Determining the adequacy of resection in fragmented curettage specimens is not possible. In most other instances, determining resection margins is often not requested, because a second procedure is anticipated by the physician based on the diagnosis. Nonetheless, some physicians may request an estimate of tumor extension to the resection margins, and in fact, the occasional tumor is completely removed by deep shave biopsy or by punch biopsy procedures. Embedding the tissue in an orientation such that sections are taken in a plane perpendicular to the epidermis allows easy identification of surgical margins along the

exposed dermis. Ink the exposed dermis before sectioning specimens greater than 0.5 cm in largest dimension. In this manner, margins may be reported as free or involved in the planes of section. Bisect any specimen 0.5 cm or greater in largest dimension and at least trisect any shave biopsy specimen 1.0 cm or greater. Tissue bags or similar aids can help confine small pieces of skin.

Elliptical Specimens

Many excisional specimens are submitted as elliptical pieces of tissue because this shape leaves wounds that lie parallel to skin tension lines, allowing easy closure and good cosmesis. That said, excisional specimens can arrive in a variety of other shapes, especially from the face, based on the anticipated closure. Round, triangular, and rhomboid specimens should be expected. Usually, there is some indication of how the specimen was oriented. For example, there can be a suture in one tip indicating the superior margin or ink placed on one or several surfaces of the tissue with an accompanying designation as to orientation. Note such identifiers in your gross description, and ink resection margins, including the deep margin. Use enough colors (generally the same ones used by the surgeon) to allow for accurate determination of precisely which margins are involved or free once the tissue is sectioned. In elliptical and rhomboid specimens, remove the small tips of the tissue fragments and place them in separate cassettes if specimen orientation is provided; one cassette may be used in the absence of anatomic identifi-

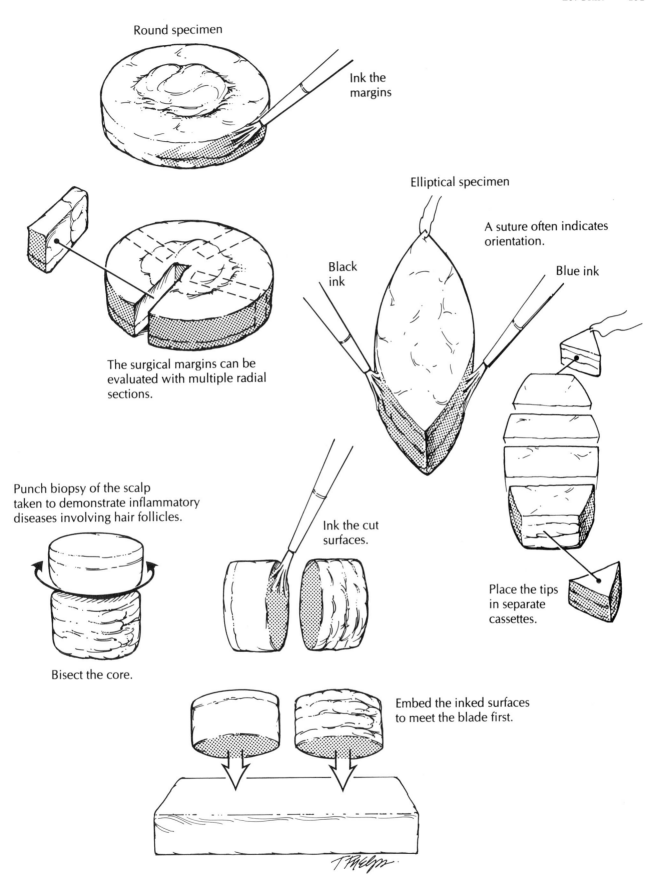

Round specimen

Ink the margins

The surgical margins can be evaluated with multiple radial sections.

Elliptical specimen

A suture often indicates orientation.

Black ink

Blue ink

Punch biopsy of the scalp taken to demonstrate inflammatory diseases involving hair follicles.

Ink the cut surfaces.

Place the tips in separate cassettes.

Bisect the core.

Embed the inked surfaces to meet the blade first.

ers. Embed the cut surface of the tip (i.e., not the surgical margin) in the block such that tissue sections progress toward the tip and become smaller over multiple tissue levels. In this way, residual tumor may be traced out into the tip. The body of the specimen can then be serially sectioned perpendicular to the epidermis in sections of roughly a nickel's width. Multiple tissue sections may be placed in single cassettes, but when necessary, single slices can be placed in cassettes to allow for more accurate determination of the location of resection margins involved with tumor. Most specimens may be submitted entirely in this fashion. Larger resections for melanoma require sampling of the margins based on visual identification of where the tumor is (was) located. In this instance, multiple samples taken perpendicular to the margin of resection and including the tumor (or biopsy wound) are recommended. The deep subcutaneous margin may have to be sampled separately.

Round Specimens

Small round excisional specimens, generally from the forehead, are a challenge. If the surgeon places an identifier on the tissue, use this information to localize the other resection margins. Because no tips are present to remove, one approach to these specimens is to tangentially shave a small piece of tissue and embed these shaves as described previously for tips from elliptical specimens, with subsequent serial slicing of the remaining tissue. The tips of elliptical specimens are generally separated from the tumor by a reliable amount of uninvolved skin. This safe zone is absent in round specimens where tumor may be close to all margins. An alternative approach is, therefore, to obtain numerous sections in radial configuration, but visualization of all margins is more difficult with this approach.

Irregularly Shaped Specimens

A similar problem arises in determining adequacy of resection margins at the base of triangular specimens. The base of such specimens generally abuts some cosmetically sensitive structure such as the eyebrow or tragus. It is difficult to determine if a margin is clear of tumor in sections taken parallel to the base of the triangle if the tumor is near the resection margin. On the other hand, perpendicular sections may miss a positive margin in the remaining tissue sections. The most reliable approach is to pay scrupulous attention to the gross appearance of the tumor and its relationship to the margins when dissecting round and triangular excisional specimens from the skin.

Punch Biopsy

The most popular method of skin sampling in the evaluation of inflammatory skin conditions is the punch or trephine biopsy. A core of tissue is obtained in this manner. Epidermis, dermis, and subcutis are usually easy to identify, and the specimen should be embedded such that tissue sections are obtained perpendicular to the plane of the epidermis. Punch biopsy specimens greater than 0.4 cm in diameter should generally be bisected. *Read the clinical history carefully!* If the clinician suspects an infectious agent, requesting appropriate special stains at the time tissue is submitted for histology will greatly shorten the time it takes to diagnose a case. Dermatophyte infection is the most commonly overlooked clinical and histologic diagnosis in the skin; obtaining fungal stains prospectively is never a waste of time or money. Certain skin conditions display only subtle or focal histologic findings, and serial sectioning of the block may be required to identify these processes, especially if a 6-mm punch biopsy specimen is submitted from a 1- or 2-mm clinical lesion. Examples include folliculitis, dermatitis herpetiformis, and transient acantholytic dermatosis.

Punch Biopsies of the Scalp

Increasingly, dermatopathologists prefer to interpret punch biopsy specimens from the scalp, taken to diagnose inflammatory conditions, in sections parallel to the plane of the epidermis. Perpendicular sectioning results in the identification of few hair follicles in a given tissue section, and then the hair follicles are only partially seen. Parallel sectioning is performed as follows. Bisect the core of tissue in a plane horizontal to the epidermis at a level approximately 1 mm above (i.e., toward the epidermis) the junction of the dermis and subcutis. Ink and embed the cut surfaces such that the inked surfaces face the microtome blade first. The tissue is serially sectioned with all tissue placed on slides. We stain every other slide to reduce the overall number of slides examined as well as to provide unstained slides for fungal stains if indicated after an initial inspection of the tissue. This method allows all follicles at a given depth in the skin to be examined in one tissue section. Examination of serial sections allows the complete assessment of follicles and follicular units contained in the core of tissue. Determination of interface changes at the epidermis (e.g., for lupus erythematosus) is generally still possible despite the horizontal sectioning, but identification of epidermal atrophy is nearly impossible. Embedded as described above, the series of slides provides sections from two pieces of tissue with progression toward the epidermis in one piece and toward the deep margin (hopefully subcutis) in the other.

Other Specimens

Dermatologic surgeons may submit somewhat untraditional specimens. Liposuction specimens consist of a variable volume of fat and serosanguineous fluid. While such specimens may be submitted as a "gross only," always examine a representative amount of fat to reduce the chances of missing the unsuspected superficial liposarcoma.

Specimens From Moh's Micrographic Surgery

A complete description of the Moh's micrographic technique of histologically controlled cutaneous surgery is beyond the scope of this chapter. In brief, after tumor debulking, wafer-thin planes of tissue are obtained from the wound bed in a horizontal orientation to the epidermis. The surgeon then carefully marks the fresh tissue to establish resection margins and to identify position in the wound bed. A map of the tissue and markings is drawn. The tissue is divided and mounted for frozen sections. The surgeon examines these sections while the patient remains in the operating suite, and the wound is still anesthetized. Identification of tumor at a resection margin prompts removal of another plane of tissue only in the involved area(s) and so on until complete removal of tumor is ensured. This technique offers a higher cure rate than conventional procedures and is tissue sparing. Based on the surgeon's routine, frozen tissue sections are placed on the slide such that tissue nearest the resection margin can be identified. Pathologists can become involved in this procedure in three ways. First, the dermatologic surgeon may seek a second opinion regarding the presence or absence of tumor in a particular frozen section. Second, a review of the frozen section slides may be requested if there is a perceived discrepancy with the biopsy diagnosis. Third, in rural areas, dermatologists will perform a similar modified technique, so-called "slow Moh's." Here, planes of skin are submitted as fixed tissue from a similarly prepared wound bed. The tissue must be processed in horizontal sections and an effort made to provide anatomic localization of involved margins based on information provided by the clinician. In the face of positive margins, the clinician will reanesthetize the (now granulating) wound base and obtain another plane of tissue. Success in this endeavor requires exceptionally good communication between the clinician, pathologist, and laboratory personnel.

Important Issues to Address in Your Surgical Pathology Report on Melanomas

- What procedure was performed, and what structures/organs are present? Specifically, record the components present (e.g., skin, subcutaneous tissue, and other soft tissue such as muscle or nerve).
- What is the histologic type of the tumor?
- What is the growth phase?
- What is the deepest level of penetration of the tumor (confined to the epidermis, into the

papillary dermis, filling the papillary dermis, into the reticular dermis, into the subcutaneous tissue)?

- What is the maximum tumor thickness? (Measure from the top of the granular layer to the deepest extent of the tumor.)
- Are any margins involved by tumor?

- How many mitotic figures are identified per square millimeter?
- Are any precursor lesions identified?
- Is any evidence of regression of the lesion present?
- Is any host inflammatory response to the tumor present?

VI The Breast

21 Breast

General Comments

A wide variety of surgical techniques are employed to biopsy or resect breast tissue. In general, these specimens can be divided into three groups: (1) small biopsies for mammographic abnormalities; (2) larger biopsies or lumpectomies; and (3) mastectomies with or without a lymph node dissection. Regardless of the type of specimen, remember that all breast tissue, even if removed for cosmetic reasons, should be examined when it is fresh.

Biopsies for Mammographic Abnormalities

Nonpalpable lesions detected mammographically are often biopsied by the surgeon and then sent to radiology, where a specimen radiograph is taken to confirm that the surgeon has indeed biopsied the lesion detected in the clinical mammogram. In these cases, the radiologist frequently will mark the lesion with a needle or dye, and the biopsy and the specimen mammogram are then brought to the surgical pathology laboratory.

As illustrated, the specimen should be inked and serially sectioned. Take care to slice the breast thinly (2 mm). Although each laboratory has its own way of designating blocks, it is important that the block containing the tissue from the area of the needle be designated. For example, we like to designate the section that contains the needle or dye as "N" and then label the adjacent sections to the left and to the right of the needle or dye sequentially as LA, LB, etc. and RA, RB, etc. Take advantage of the specimen radiograph; the gross findings can be correlated with the lesion seen radiographically. Also, note the largest dimension of the lesion. If the grossly detectable tumor is large enough for a portion to be submitted for estrogen and progesterone receptor analysis (generally larger than 1 cm), first confirm that the tissue submitted is cancerous with a frozen section, or a fine-needle aspirate. If an invasive carcinoma is identified, then submit a fresh, appropriately sized portion of the carcinoma for estrogen and progesterone receptor analysis and for ploidy studies (Table 21-1). Carefully note the relationship of the tumor to the inked margins as well as the circumscription and nature of the border of the tumor. When a tumor is grossly identified, submit at least three sections of the tumor and extensively sample the adjacent breast tissue, including the inked margins. Again, in taking these sections, be sure to take sections that demonstrate the relation of the tumor to the inked margin. If no tumor is identified, submit the entire specimen, up to 16 blocks of tissue, for histological examination.

In evaluating these biopsies histologically, it is very important to note the type, grade, and size of any neoplasm and its relationship to the margins. If no tumor is present, document that the surgeon has removed the mammographically suspicious lesion (i.e. calcifications or a density) and that the mammographic lesion has been histologically evaluated. For example, if a biopsy is performed for microcalcifications, these calcifications should be identified microscopically.

Biopsy

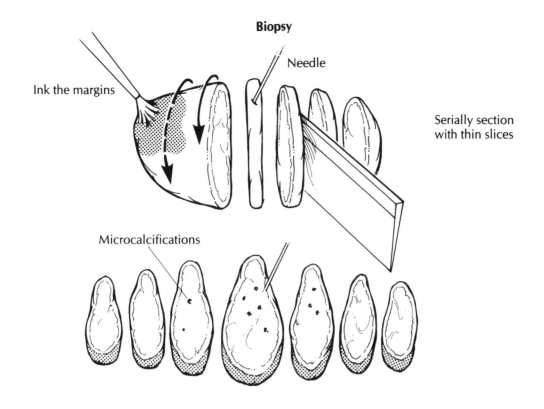

Ink the margins

Needle

Serially section with thin slices

Microcalcifications

Lumpectomy

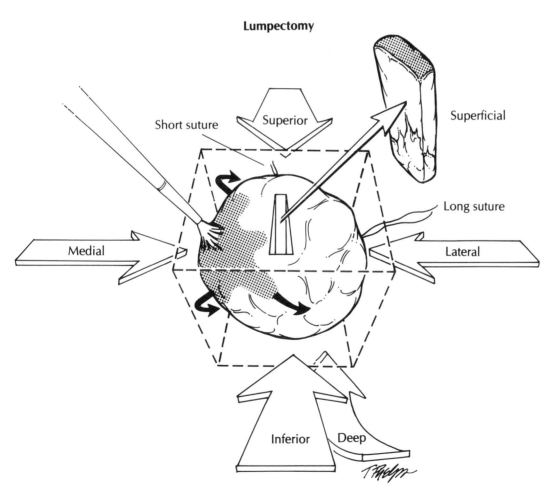

Short suture

Superior

Superficial

Medial

Long suture

Lateral

Inferior

Deep

TABLE 21-1. Submission of breast tumors for hormone receptor analysis.

- Process the specimen before it is fixed so that the fresh tumor can be sampled and submitted. Avoid unnecessary delays in collecting the tumor sample.
- Submit an adequate sample. Although requirements vary from laboratory to laboratory, in general, most hormone receptor assays and additional ancillary studies (e.g., ploidy and S-phase analysis) can be performed on 1 g of tissue. Make sure you are familiar with the requirements of your laboratory.
- Quickly freeze the tumor sample in liquid nitrogen, then place it in an appropriately labeled container for storage and transport.
- Do not collect the tumor if it is too small. Likewise, do not sample the tumor from an area where it approaches a surgical margin. The submission of a breast tumor for hormone receptor analysis should never compromise the pathologist's ability to establish the diagnosis and evaluate the adequacy of excision.

Larger Biopsies/Lumpectomies for Grossly Identifiable Tumors

Larger biopsies are usually brought directly to the surgical pathology laboratory. Frequently, but not universally, the surgeon will orient the specimen by placing a short stitch in the superior aspect of the specimen and a long stitch in the lateral aspect of the specimen. Since you know which breast the biopsy was taken from (left or right), these landmarks can be used to identify all of the other margins. As illustrated, these margins are easier to conceptualize if you think of the specimen as a cube. After orienting the specimen, ink it and take perpendicular sections from all six margins (superior, inferior, medial, lateral, superficial, and deep). Examine the specimen in the manner described above for the smaller biopsies. In addition, if a portion of skin is present, it can help orient the specimen, and it should also be inked and sampled for histological examination.

Mastectomies

True radical mastectomies are now seldom performed. This procedure includes a complete axillary dissection including removal of the pectoralis major and minor muscles. More com-
monly, a modified radical mastectomy is performed. In this procedure, the undersurface of the specimen is composed only of fascial planes with occasional shreds of pectoralis major muscle attached. Nevertheless, a complete axillary dissection typically is attached to the breast forming an elongated tail at one end of the otherwise elliptical specimen. Most mastectomies are performed after an open biopsy; however, occasionally, a diagnosis is made by aspiration or needle biopsy. If tissue for ploidy analysis and estrogen and progesterone receptor studies was not submitted from the original biopsy, fresh tissue from the primary tumor within the mastectomy should be sent for these studies (see Table 21-1). This tissue should be submitted as soon as possible after receiving the specimen. If the primary tumor is not available, then portions of large lymph node metastases also may be used for receptor studies. Once tissue for receptor studies has been obtained, the remaining mastectomy tissues may be handled in a more leisurely manner.

First, orient the specimen to correctly localize the four quadrants of the breast. Typically, this procedure should not be difficult. Use the axillary contents, the side (left or right) from which the breast was taken, and the surgeon's description of the location of the tumor and biopsy site to orient the specimen. Once the specimen has been oriented, place a safety pin in the corner of the upper outer quadrant. This will help you to reorient the specimen quickly in case you ever have to return to the specimen. The axillary tail can then be removed for later examination. Next, take the time to palpate the specimen. Localize the biopsy scar, the biopsy cavity, and any masses. Examine the deep surface of the specimen for attached fragments of skeletal muscle. If this deep surface is puckered and indurated, ink it so that perpendicular sections can be taken to evaluate the deep soft tissue margin. The breast can then be placed skin surface down on a cutting board and sectioned. As illustrated, use the nipple to center the specimen, and then with two long perpendicular cuts, section the breast into four quadrants. Each quadrant can then be further sectioned, each in its own direction. These cuts should not go all the way through the specimen, but instead should leave the pieces attached together by a thin rim of unsectioned breast or skin. This

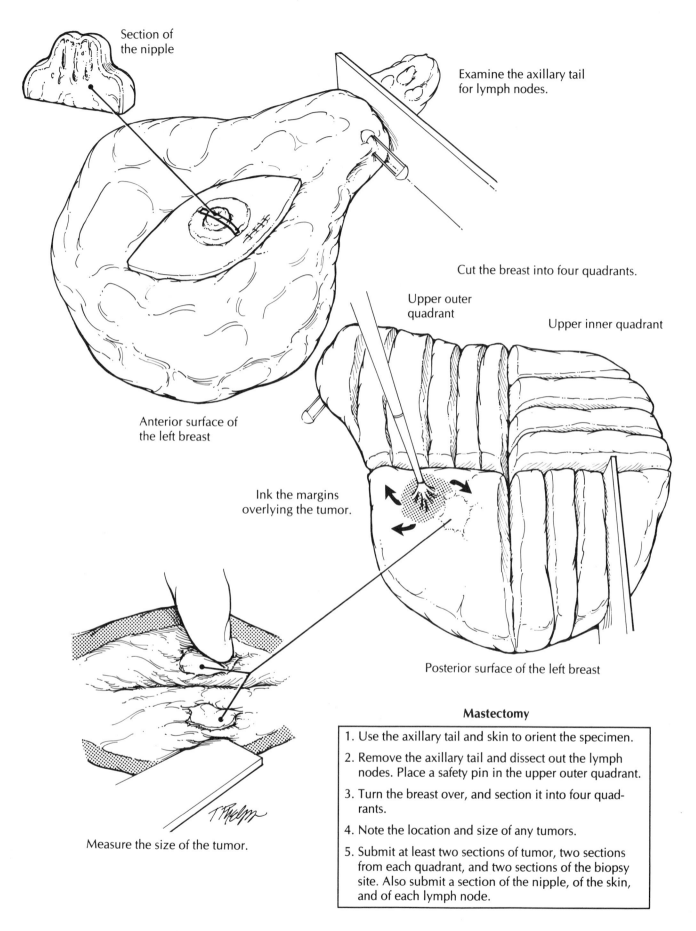

Section of the nipple

Examine the axillary tail for lymph nodes.

Cut the breast into four quadrants.

Upper outer quadrant

Upper inner quadrant

Anterior surface of the left breast

Ink the margins overlying the tumor.

Posterior surface of the left breast

Measure the size of the tumor.

Mastectomy

1. Use the axillary tail and skin to orient the specimen.

2. Remove the axillary tail and dissect out the lymph nodes. Place a safety pin in the upper outer quadrant.

3. Turn the breast over, and section it into four quadrants.

4. Note the location and size of any tumors.

5. Submit at least two sections of tumor, two sections from each quadrant, and two sections of the biopsy site. Also submit a section of the nipple, of the skin, and of each lymph node.

procedure not only will help orient the specimen but will also help remind you to document which quadrant(s) the lesion is in.

The gross description should include: (1) the overall dimensions and the weight of the specimen; (2) the overall dimensions of the skin surface; (3) the presence or absence of a biopsy scar and biopsy cavity, and their relationship to the nipple; (4) the presence of any retraction or ulceration of the nipple and/or surrounding skin; (5) the presence or absence of muscle on the undersurface of the specimen; and finally, (6) *the size and gross appearance of the tumor including the quadrant of the breast in which it is localized.* At least two sections of the breast primary should be submitted for histologic examination. If a biopsy was performed at an earlier date, at least two sections from the biopsy site should be submitted, including any suspicious areas of induration. Two sections can then be submitted from each of the remaining breast quadrants to include any focal lesions. If the mastectomy was performed as a prophylactic procedure in a patient with an *in situ* carcinoma, submit at least three sections from each quadrant. Also, submit a section of the nipple and of the skin. Then dissect all lymph nodes from the axillary contents. Section the nodes, note any gross abnormalities, and submit a representative section of each node. Because axillary levels are determined by their relationship to the pectoralis minor muscle, it is impossible to state the levels of the axillary contents with certainty unless the surgeon designates these levels. If the levels are not designated, only the total node counts are important.

Important Issues to Address in Your Surgical Pathology Report on Breast Biopsies and Resections

- What procedure was performed, and what structures/organs are present?

- Are microcalcifications present?
- What are the size and location (nipple, central portion, upper inner quadrant, upper outer quadrant, lower inner quadrant, lower outer quadrant, axillary tail) of any tumors identified?
- Are the tumors in situ or infiltrating?
- What are the histologic type and grade of any neoplasms identified?
- Is vascular/lymphatic invasion present?
- Is the skin or nipple involved?
- Does the tumor involve the margins of resection? Does it extend directly into the chest wall?
- Record the location and number of nodes examined and the presence or absence of metastatic carcinoma in these nodes. How large is the largest metastasis? Is there extranodal extension of the carcinoma?

Breast Implants

The handling of prosthetic breast implants deserves special note: We suggest that you follow The College of American Pathologists (CAP) recommendations.[3] Briefly, they suggest that you first weigh the implant. Then describe its external surface (smooth, textured, etc.); its contents (clear gel, oil, or watery fluid); and its condition (intact or ruptured). Next, document any inscriptions printed on the implant, and photograph the implant, particularly if it is ruptured. You can then turn your attention to the tissue capsule—the wall of fibroconnective tissue that forms around the breast implant. Weigh and measure the capsule, describe its inner surface, and submit one to two tissue sections of the capsule for histology. If any nodules are present in the capsule, they should be sampled more extensively. Finally, store the implants. With the current flood of litigation, the implants should probably be stored indefinitely.

VII   The Female Genital System

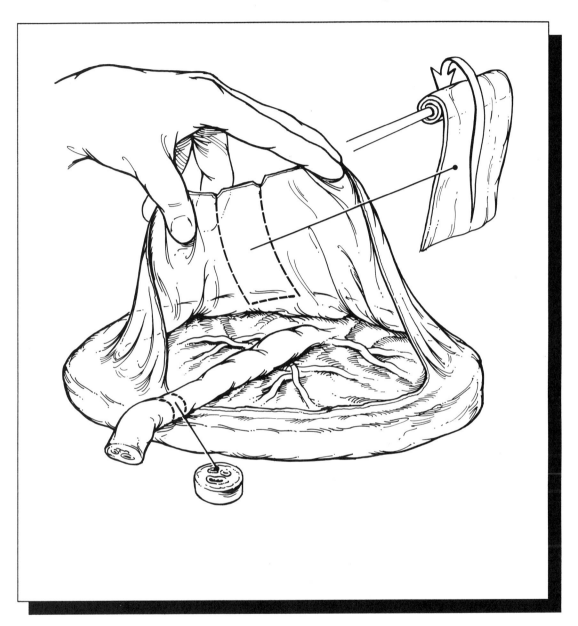

22 Vulva

General Comments

The *vulva* collectively refers to the external female genitalia. It includes the mons pubis, labia majora and minora, clitoris, vestibule with the urethral and vaginal orifices, posterior fourchette and perineum. The epithelial covering is predominately skin (keratinized, stratified squamous epithelium), except for the vestibule, which is mucosa (nonkeratinized). Vulvar diseases are primarily epithelial in origin and usually can be seen externally. Therefore, most vulvar specimens can be handled in a manner similar to other skin specimens with emphasis on proper orientation and an evaluation of surgical margins.

Small Biopsies

Diagnostic punch biopsies are usually performed for lesions that appear as unusual discolorations or thickenings of the vulva. The most important tasks are to orient the specimen so that sections will be taken perpendicular to the epithelial surface and to secure the specimen properly so that small pieces are not lost in processing. When multiple sites have been biopsied to map out the extent of a lesion, be sure to clearly designate each separate location in the diagnosis.

Cavitronic Ultrasonic Surgical Aspirator (CUSA) Biopsies

A CUSA can be used for the treatment of condyloma acuminata and vulvar intraepithelial neoplasia (VIN). This technique simultaneously disrupts tissue by ultrasound and aspirates tissue. Numerous small fragments of epithelium with little or no underlying stroma are generated. Due to the size and quantity of the fragments, orientation of the epithelial surface is not possible. The best approach is to handle these tissues like a curettage specimen. First, collect all the tissue fragments by pouring the contents of the specimen container through a filter. Next, submit the tissue as an aggregate either within a fine-mesh biopsy bag or wrapped in tissue paper. Multiple levels can then be ordered on each tissue block to assist with the three-dimensional orientation of the lesion.

Excisional Biopsies

Excisional biopsies of the vulva range from simple excisions of inclusion cysts to wide local excisions of premalignant lesions or minimally invasive cancers. The tissue submitted usually consists of an ellipse of skin with a variable amount of underlying soft tissue and it often lacks any identifiable anatomic landmarks. Look for a stitch or diagram provided by the gynecologist for orientation. It is crucial not to proceed with the dissection until you understand the *in situ* configuration of the specimen. These specimens can be handled in the same way as other excisional biopsies of skin (see Chapter 20). Ink all the margins (both cutaneous and deep) and take sections perpendicular to the epithelial surface. The separate cutaneous margins should be clearly designated. Be prepared to submit the entire specimen in order to rule out or confirm invasive disease and to document the adequacy of the resection margins.

Vulvectomies

The majority of vulvectomies are performed for the treatment of invasive squamous carcinoma. Most squamous carcinomas arise on the labia

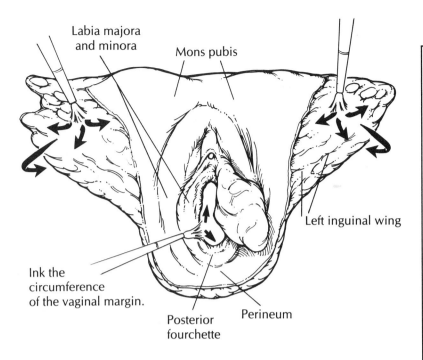

Labia majora and minora

Mons pubis

Left inguinal wing

Ink the circumference of the vaginal margin.

Posterior fourchette

Perineum

Total Vulvectomy

1. Orient the specimen as if viewed in situ with the inguinal wings superior and lateral.

2. Ink all cutaneous and soft tissue margins, including the deep margin. Ink the vaginal margin with a separate color.

3. Document the size of all lesions and section with full-thickness incisions perpendicular to the epithelial surface.

4. Dissect the inguinal wings for lymph nodes and maintain their right and left orientation.

5. Submit sections of tumor to demonstrate maximum tumor thickness; nearest margins (vaginal, cutaneous, and deep); any other skin lesions; all lymph nodes; and uninvolved skin including clitoris, fourchette, perineum, and contralateral labia majora and minora.

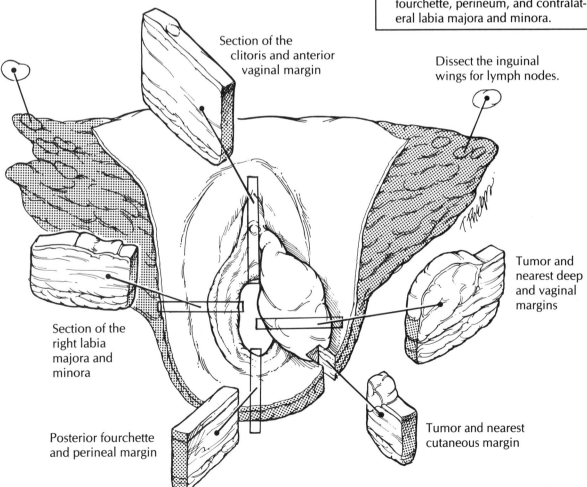

Section of the clitoris and anterior vaginal margin

Dissect the inguinal wings for lymph nodes.

Tumor and nearest deep and vaginal margins

Section of the right labia majora and minora

Posterior fourchette and perineal margin

Tumor and nearest cutaneous margin

(usually the labia majora), with the remainder primarily located on either the clitoris or posterior fourchette. Vulvectomy specimens can be either partial—when only a portion of the vulva is removed—or total—when the whole vulvar region is removed. A portion of the vagina and extensions of perineum around the anus may also be included. The depth of the resection is variable. A *superficial vulvectomy* refers to the removal of the epidermis with a variable amount of dermis and subcutaneous tissue. A *deep vulvectomy* refers to removal of the vulva to the superficial aponeurosis of the urogenital diaphragm and/or pubic periosteum. Inguinal node dissections can either be attached to the vulvectomy specimen as superolateral wings or submitted separately.

The initial evaluation includes orientation and documentation of the tissues received. Begin by orienting the specimen as if viewed *in situ*. With a total vulvectomy, this is easily accomplished by placing the inguinal fat superiorly and laterally. If the inguinal region is not present, use the clitoris to define the superior and midline position. In partial vulvectomies, orient the specimen using the hair-bearing labia majora, which represents the lateral extent of the resection. If there is any doubt, ask the surgeon to help with orientation. Document the type of specimen received and the anatomic structures present. Measure the width of the specimen, the length from the superior to inferior limits, and the depth from the epithelial surface to the deep soft tissue margin. It may be helpful to have photographs, line drawings, or preprinted diagrams to demonstrate the margins of resection and extent of the lesion. Ink all the exposed epithelial and soft tissue margins. The vaginal margin should be painted with a different color ink than the other cutaneous margins. The specimen can then be pinned to a cork or wax board for fixation.

After fixation, examine the epithelial surface for ulcerative, exophytic, and flat lesions. Evaluate all lesions with full-thickness incisions perpendicular to the epithelial surface. Record their location, size, and distance to the nearest skin and vaginal margins. For invasive tumors, also measure the maximal tumor thickness and the distance from the deepest tumor edge to the nearest deep margin. Submit sections of the tumor in such a way as to include the nearest deep and epithelial (both vaginal and cutaneous) margins as well as adjacent normal-appearing skin. Preneoplastic lesions such as vulvar intraepithelial neoplasia (VIN) may be found adjacent to tumors. Margins should be evaluated with sections that are perpendicular rather than parallel to the surgical margin. Representative epithelial margins distant to the tumor do not need to be submitted. Judiciously sample any other skin lesions, especially those within 0.5 cm of any margin. Include sections of non-neoplastic skin so that it can be evaluated for the presence of lichen sclerosus, squamous hyperplasia, and hyperkeratosis.

In vulvectomy specimens with attached inguinal regions, the lymph nodes can be dissected either before or after obtaining the appropriate epithelial sections. Turn the specimen over so that the epithelial surface is face down and the subcutaneous tissue is exposed. Beginning at the superior tip of one inguinal wing, and progressing medially, make parallel 0.3- to 0.4-cm-wide sections through the fatty tissue. Examine the cut fat carefully for lymph nodes. Although the lymphatic drainage of the vulva can be divided into superficial and deep node groups, this is usually not necessary and important nodes, such as Cloquet's node, must be separately designated by the surgeon. All the lymph nodes should be entirely submitted unless grossly positive, in which case a representative section will suffice. Be sure to clearly designate and submit the right and left node groups separately.

Important Issues to Address in Your Surgical Pathology Report on Vulvectomies

- What type of vulvectomy was performed (partial vs. total, superficial vs. deep), and what structures are present?
- Where is the tumor located? Is it unifocal or multifocal?
- What is the size of the tumor (in centimeters)?
- What are the histologic type and grade of the neoplasm?
- What is the "maximum tumor thickness" (in millimeters)? (Measure from the granular layer if keratinized or surface if nonkeratinized.)
- What is the "maximum depth of invasion" (in millimeters)? (Measure from the epithelial stromal junction of the adjacent most superficial dermal papillae.)
- Does the tumor involve any of the margins? (vaginal, cutaneous, or deep)?
- Does the tumor extend into any adjacent tissues (lower urethra, upper urethra, vagina, anus, bladder, or rectum)?
- Is there evidence of lymphatic, vascular, or perineural invasion?
- Does the adjacent skin show any associated squamous changes (VIN or squamous hyperplasia)?
- Does the tumor involve the inguinal lymph nodes? (Include the number of nodes involved and the number of nodes examined separately on each side.)
- Does the non-neoplastic portion of the vulva show any pathology?

23 Uterus, Cervix, and Vagina

Biopsies

Cervical and vaginal biopsies consist of an epithelial surface and varying amounts of underlying stroma. Usually, no grossly identifiable lesion can be seen. The most important objectives are to orient the specimen so that perpendicular sections will be taken through the surface and to secure the specimen properly to ensure that small pieces are not lost. These tasks can be accomplished in several ways. If the specimen is large enough (i.e., greater than 0.4 cm), the tissue can be bisected perpendicular to the surface and marked with either mercurochrome or tattoo powder to indicate the surface to be cut. If the specimen is small, it can be secured between Gelfoam sponges, within fine-mesh biopsy bags, or it can be wrapped in tissue paper. The gynecologist may also submit the biopsy oriented mucosal side up on a mounting surface such as filter paper. In this case, instruct your histotechnologist to embed and cut the biopsy specimen perpendicular to the mounting surface. All biopsy specimens should be entirely submitted, and it is often useful to routinely request that multiple levels be performed by the histology laboratory.

Endometrial biopsies should be handled similarly to curettage specimens.

Curettings

Endocervical and endometrial curettings consist of multiple small fragments of epithelium, which are often admixed with blood and mucus. The surgeon may put the curettings on Telfa pads or directly into fixative. Scrape the Telfa pad carefully on both sides, and filter the fluid of the specimen container into a tissue bag to obtain all tissue fragments. Record the aggregate dimension, and note the percentage of tissue versus the percentage of blood and mucus. The entire specimen should be submitted either wrapped in tissue paper or within a fine-mesh biopsy bag. Even if no tissue is visible, the blood and mucus should still be submitted for histologic evaluation, as they may contain entrapped small epithelial fragments. Multiple levels are often useful in evaluating these specimens.

Cervix

Loop Electrocautery Excisions

The loop electrosurgical excision procedure (LEEP) and large loop excision of the transformation zone (LLETZ) are electrocautery excisions of the cervical transformation zone that excise less tissue than the traditional cone biopsy. Their use is increasing in the treatment of squamous intraepithelial lesions. Depending on the type of loop used and on the depth of the excision, the specimen may be large enough to allow one to orient, open, and process it like a conventional cone biopsy, as described later. However, many of these specimens arrive in the surgical pathology laboratory already fixed in formalin and/or in several pieces. The endocervical margin will sometimes be submitted separately, and an overall orientation may or may not be provided. If multiple fragments are submitted, identify the mucosal surface, and try to

Loop Electrocautery Excisions of the Cervix

1. Orient the specimen by identifying the ectocervical and endocervical margins.
2. Ink the endocervical margin and the stromal/ectocervical margins with separate colors.
3. For small cylindrical specimens, divide in half and section longitudinally.
4. For shallow, saucer-shaped specimens, section radially—like a pie.
5. Submit the entire specimen.

Square large loop electrosurgical instrument

Endocervical margin

Stroma

Cervical canal

Ectocervical margin

Section longitudinally

Hemispheric loop electrosurgical instrument

Cervical canal

Ectocervical margin

Stroma

Section radially

discern the smooth, gray squamous mucosa from the rugated, mucoid, tan endocervical mucosa. Divide the fragments into strips with sections perpendicular to the squamocolumnar junction. For shallow, saucer-shaped specimens, divide the specimen radially as illustrated. This is similar to slicing a pie. For small conical specimens that are already well fixed, divide the specimen into anterior and posterior halves, and section each half longitudinally as shown. Conceptually, cutting the biopsy this way is similar to the handling of the perpendicular sections of the distal urethral margins in a radical prostatectomy specimen. Note that in contrast to large cone biopsies, not all sections will demonstrate the cervical canal mucosa. Although cautery artifact may make the limits of resection of these specimens difficult to evaluate, it is always best to ink the mucosal margins and exposed stroma for histologic evaluation.

Cone Biopsy

A cervical cone biopsy is a conical excision of the cervical canal performed with either a laser or surgical blade (cold knife excision). The wider part of the cone is the outer ectocervix, and the tapered end is the endocervical margin. By convention, the ectocervix is described as a clock face with the most superior midpoint of the anterior lip designated as 12 o'clock. This point is usually marked with a stitch by the gynecologist. After orienting the cone biopsy as if viewed *in situ*, ink the exposed fibrous stroma and the ectocervical mucosal margin. Use a different color to ink the endocervical mucosal margin. Make a longitudinal incision through the outer stroma to the inner canal at the 3-o'clock position, and open the specimen so that the inner mucosal surface is exposed. The convention of incising the cervix at either 3 or 9 o'clock is based on the fact that most cervical lesions arise on the anterior and posterior surfaces, rather than laterally. Pin the specimen to either a wax or cork board with the epithelial surface upward, using pins placed through the stroma on both sides. Examine the mucosal surface, and look for any lesions, especially along the squamocolumnar junction.

After fixation, cut serial full-thickness sections perpendicular to the mucosal surface in the plane of the endocervical canal. Use the en-

docervical apex as a pivot, and angle the cuts to provide a continuous line from the endocervical mucosa to the ectocervical mucosa. These cuts will encompass the squamocolumnar junction and will demonstrate the extent of the transformation zone. The sections should be 0.2 to 0.3 cm wide and will end up being slightly wedge shaped. All sections should be submitted and designated as to their clock-face orientation. As with other biopsies, multiple levels are often routinely requested.

Important Issues to Address in Your Surgical Pathology Report on the Cervix

- What procedure was performed, and what structures/organs are present?
- What grade of squamous intraepithelial lesion is identified?
- Is the lesion focal, multifocal, or extensive?
- Are the resection margins involved (endocervical, ectocervical or stromal)?
- Is evidence of invasion present? If so, what is the depth of invasion from the basement membrane (in millimeters)? What is the maximum linear width (in millimeters)? Is there any evidence of capillary–lymphatic space invasion?

Uterus

The uterus is removed for a wide variety of reasons. Common indications for hysterectomy include uterine prolapse, leiomyomas, endometrial hyperplasia, cervical cancer, and endometrial cancer. Given the diverse nature of these processes, and the variation in the appearance of the uterus due to the hormonal environment, it is important to know both the clinical indication for the surgery and the patient's reproductive status when evaluating a hysterectomy specimen.

The uterus is traditionally divided into two components: (1) the uterine corpus and (2) the uterine cervix. The uterine corpus (or body) extends from the superiorly located fundus to the point of maximal narrowing which corresponds to the location of the internal os. The right and left cornual regions are located superolaterally,

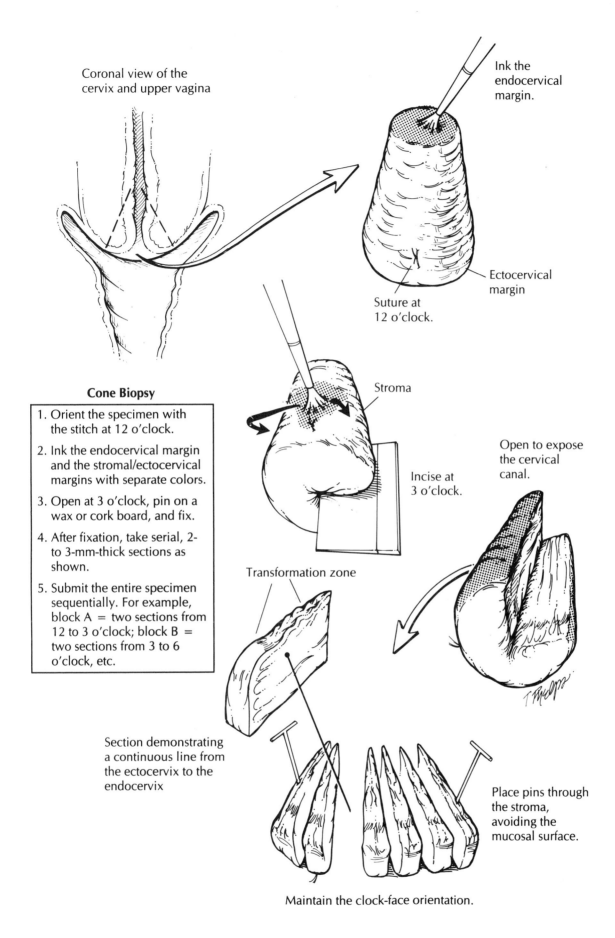

Coronal view of the cervix and upper vagina

Ink the endocervical margin.

Ectocervical margin

Suture at 12 o'clock.

Stroma

Incise at 3 o'clock.

Open to expose the cervical canal.

Cone Biopsy

1. Orient the specimen with the stitch at 12 o'clock.

2. Ink the endocervical margin and the stromal/ectocervical margins with separate colors.

3. Open at 3 o'clock, pin on a wax or cork board, and fix.

4. After fixation, take serial, 2- to 3-mm-thick sections as shown.

5. Submit the entire specimen sequentially. For example, block A = two sections from 12 to 3 o'clock; block B = two sections from 3 to 6 o'clock, etc.

Transformation zone

Section demonstrating a continuous line from the ectocervix to the endocervix

Place pins through the stroma, avoiding the mucosal surface.

Maintain the clock-face orientation.

at the insertion of the fallopian tubes. The inferior 1 to 2 cm of the corpus is referred to as the isthmus or lower uterine segment (LUS). This region is a "bridge" between the cervix and the uterus and demonstrates a gradual transition from endocervical to endometrial mucosa. The cervix encompasses the lower portion of the uterus, beginning at the internal os. The cervix is composed of an inner endocervical canal lined by columnar epithelium and a rounded outer ectocervix covered by squamous epithelium. The location of the squamocolumnar junction moves in and out of the cervical canal with age and parity. It is within this region that most intraepithelial lesions arise. Although the exact limits of this region are not visible grossly, the term "transformation zone" encompasses this entire transition area including the squamocolumnar junction.

This section provides an approach to the evaluation of hysterectomy specimens in four categories: (1) hysterectomies for nonmalignant disease, (2) hysterectomies for endometrial cancer, (3) radical hysterectomies for cervical cancer, and (4) pelvic exenterations with vaginectomies for vaginal cancer or recurrent cervical cancer.

Hysterectomy for Nonmalignant Disease

The category of hysterectomy of nonmalignant disease includes hysterectomies for uterine prolapse, persistent abnormal bleeding, intractable pelvic pain, leiomyomas, and endometrial hyperplasia. The procedure can be performed either vaginally or abdominally. The fallopian tubes and ovaries may also be present.

Orient the uterus by identifying the stubs of the round ligaments that insert anterior to the fallopian tubes. The ovaries should lie posteriorly. In addition, because the anterior peritoneum reflects onto the bladder, the anterior peritoneum does not extend as far inferiorly along the uterus as does the posterior peritoneum. Vaginal and abdominal hysterectomies may be distinguished by examining the peritoneal surface in the region of the posterior cul-de-sac. The peritoneum appears V-shaped in a vaginal and U-shaped in an abdominal hysterectomy specimen.

If the adnexa are present, remove them from the right and left cornual regions, and examine them separately (see Chapter 24). Weigh the uterus, and record the following measurements: fundus to ectocervix, cornu to cornu, and anterior to posterior. Measure the length of the cervix from the level of the internal os to the ectocervix and the diameter of the cervix from side to side and from anterior to posterior.

The uterus can now be evaluated with a systematic examination of each of its main components. Begin by examining the uterine serosa. Look for and describe any adhesions or small "powder burn" spots, which may signify endometriosis. These may be seen more frequently on the posterior aspect.

Next, evaluate the cervix. Note the shape of the external os, which is usually circular in nulliparous women and slit-like in parous women. Examine the ectocervix for any lacerations, scars, masses, ulcers, or cysts. Place a probe through the cervical canal and into the endometrial cavity. Beginning at the cervix, incise the uterus with a large blade using the probe as a guide to divide it into anterior and posterior halves. Gently remove the excess mucus from the endocervical canal, and examine it for the presence of polyps. At this point, the uterus may be photographed and then pinned to a wax tablet for fixation. Be sure to avoid placing pins through the mucosal surfaces. After fixation, longitudinally section the cervix at 0.2- to 0.3-cm intervals, and evaluate the transformation zone and stroma.

Now, measure the thickness of the endometrium, and look for any unusual thickenings or polyps. Keep in mind the age and reproductive status of the patient. If the woman is postmenopausal, an endometrial thickness greater than 2 mm may signify a hyperplastic process. Conversely, a thick endometrium in a premenopausal woman may reflect only the normal secretory phase.

The myometrium is examined last. Make serial 0.5-cm-thick transverse cuts through the uterine corpus and isthmus, and record the myometrial thickness. Look for intramural leiomyomas or evidence of adenomyosis. Adenomyosis is usually more extensive in the posterior wall and may be recognized by a thickened wall with trabeculations and small hemorrhagic or cystic foci.

Fallopian tube

Round ligament

Anterior extent of the peritoneum

Section of leiomyoma with adjacent myometrium

Right cornu

Fundus

Corpus

Lower uterine segment (LUS)

Internal os

Endometrium

Myometrium

Serosa

Endocervical canal

Ectocervix

Endocervical epithelium

Squamous epithelium

Longitudinal section encompassing the transformation zone

Hysterectomy for Nonmalignant Disease

1. Orient the uterus: The round ligaments are most anterior, and the ovaries, if present, are most posterior. The peritoneum extends further inferiorly along the posterior aspect of the uterus than it does anteriorly.

2. Remove adnexa, if present, and weigh and record measurements of the uterus and cervix.

3. Place a probe through the endocervical canal and into the endometrial cavity. Bivalve the uterus into anterior and posterior halves with a long blade.

4. Longitudinally section the cervix to evaluate the transformation zone.

5. Serially bread-loaf the uterine corpus and LUS with 0.5-cm transverse slices.

6. Submit one section each of the anterior and posterior cervix and one section each of the anterior and posterior endomyometrium with serosa.

7. For leiomyomata, submit representative sections of all myomas greater than 5 cm. If regions of hemorrhage, necrosis, or softening are present, then submit one section per 1 cm of tumor diameter. For squamous intraepithelial lesions, submit the entire cervix as in a cone biopsy. For endometrial hyperplasia, submit the entire endometrium.

If no lesions are identified, standard sections of the uterus include longitudinal sections of the anterior and posterior cervix (including the transformation zone) and full-thickness sections of the anterior and posterior walls of the uterus to include endometrium, myometrium, and serosa. At our institution, sections of the anterior and posterior lower uterine segment regions are routinely submitted as well.

Additional sampling may also be required if the standard sections reveal either endometrial hyperplasia or a cervical intraepithelial lesion. In the case of endometrial hyperplasia, the entire endometrium may need to be evaluated to rule out an invasive process. Multiple thin strips of endometrium with only a small amount of underlying myometrium can be submitted in a limited number of tissue cassettes. If a high-grade squamous intraepithelial lesion is identified, the cervix should be processed and submitted as described for cone biopsies. For low-grade squamous intraepithelial lesions, a section from each quadrant may suffice.

The evaluation of a uterus with multiple leiomyomas deserves special mention. A leiomyomatous uterus is one of the most frequently encountered specimens, and the gross examination of these specimens is the key to their proper handling. Orient, weigh, measure, and section the uterus as described above. Record the number of nodules present and their size. Specifically state whether they are submucosal, intramural, or subserosal in location. All nodules should be sectioned at 1- to 2-cm intervals and examined grossly but not necessarily microscopically. Benign leiomyomas are firm and white with a whorled cut surface. Their border with the surrounding myometrium is smooth and well-circumscribed. If these criteria are met, representative sampling of each leiomyoma is sufficient. Always include sections demonstrating the border between the leiomyoma and the surrounding myometrium or overlying endometrium. Any leiomyomas with areas of hemorrhage, necrosis, and softening need to be sampled more extensively. In these cases, the general rule of one section per 1 cm of tumor diameter should be followed. Smooth muscle tumors less than 5 cm do not need to be sampled, as they rarely metastasize, regardless of their microscopic appearance.

Important Issues to Address in Your Surgical Pathology Report on Hysterectomies for Non-Malignant Disease

- What procedure was performed, and what structures/organs are present?
- Cervix: Are any preinvasive or invasive lesions identified?
- Endometrium: Is the endometrium hyperplastic, atrophic, or functional? If functional, specify whether it is in the proliferative or secretory phase.
- Myometrium: Are any leiomyomas or regions of adenomyosis identified? Specify whether the leiomyomas are submucosal, intramural, or subserosal.
- Serosa: Are any adhesions or regions of endometriosis identified?

Hysterectomy for Endometrial Cancer

The approach to hysterectomies performed for endometrial cancer parallels the approach to hysterectomies for benign disease. Additional steps include inking the paracervical and parametrial soft tissue margins and evaluating the extent of the tumor.

Orient, weigh, and measure the uterus as described in the section on hysterectomies for benign disease, and ink the soft tissue resection margins around the cervical canal. Also, ink the parametrial tissue, which extends along the body of the uterus and into the broad ligament. Carefully examine the serosal surfaces for evidence of tumor extension. Ink these areas a different color for orientation. If the adnexa are present, remove them at their lateral insertions along the uterus. Make multiple transverse cuts through the ovary and fallopian tube, looking for evidence of either direct tumor extension or metastatic spread. Submit at least one section from each side to demonstrate the ovary and fallopian tube with adjacent soft tissue.

Bivalve the uterus by using a long, sharp knife guided by a probe placed through the cervical canal. Closely examine the endometrial cavity. Endometrial carcinomas can be shaggy, sessile tumors or polypoid masses arising from

Fallopian tube

Anterior aspect

Paracervical stroma

Round ligament

Parametrial tissue

Tumor

Myometrium

Section demonstrating maximum tumor thickness

Serosa

Section of tumor and adjacent endomyometrium

Endocervical canal

Section of LUS with tumor extending to the endocervix

Uterine corpus

Lower uterine segment (LUS)

Cervix

Transformation zone

Hysterectomy for Endometrial Cancer

1. Orient the uterus: The round ligaments are most anterior, and the ovaries, if present, are most posterior. The peritoneum extends further inferiorly along the posterior aspect of the uterus than it does anteriorly.

2. Weigh and measure the uterus and cervix. Ink the paracervical and parametrial soft tissue margins.

3. Place a probe in the endocervical and endometrial canal. Bivalve the uterus into anterior and posterior halves with a long blade.

4. Longitudinally section the cervix, extending the incision upward through the LUS. Serially bread-loaf the uterine corpus with 0.5-cm transverse slices.

5. Describe the size, appearance, and location of the tumor.

6. Submit sections of tumor to demonstrate the maximum tumor thickness, anterior and posterior LUS sections, uninvolved endometrium, and anterior and posterior cervix. If the adnexa are present, submit sections of the ovary and fallopian tube with adjacent soft tissue.

the surface of the endometrium. They may be either focal or diffuse. The sounding depth of the uterus from the external cervical os to the superior limit of the endometrial cavity may be measured, but it is no longer used in the staging of endometrial cancers. While the tumor is fresh, remove a portion to freeze for estrogen/progesterone receptor assays or future molecular diagnostic tests if desired. The bivalved uterus may now be photographed and pinned to a wax tablet for fixation.

The dissection begins with longitudinal sectioning of the cervix. Extend these incisions through the lower uterine segment to include both endometrial and endocervical mucosal surfaces. Note whether or not the tumor grossly involves the endocervical mucosa and/or stroma. Submit a section of this region from the anterior and posterior halves to evaluate for tumor extension into the cervix, an important factor in determining the stage of the cancer. This step may also be accomplished by taking transverse sections of the upper endocervix and lower uterine segment. Next, serially bread-loaf the uterine corpus and lower uterine segment with transverse sections. Record the size, location, and appearance of the tumor. Describe the pattern of invasion. Does the tumor have a broad pushing front, an infiltrating finger-like pattern, or is it discontinuous? Measure the greatest depth of tumor invasion into the myometrium starting from the normal junction of the endometrium and the myometrium. In addition, measure the total myometrial thickness at this point, and specify the uninvolved distance from the deep tumor/myometrial junction to the serosa. When selecting sections for histologic analysis, include the deepest point of tumor invasion as well as the interface with grossly uninvolved endometrium. The best sections are those that show the full thickness from the endometrium to the serosa. Sometimes, however, the myometrium may be too thick to fit in a standard-size tissue cassette. In these situations, divide the section into endometrial and serosal halves. Be sure to designate their relationship clearly in your summary of sections.

Lymph nodes from the pelvic and para-aortic regions may also be included as separate specimens. They can be handled in a routine manner for evaluation of metastatic disease.

Important Issues to Address in Your Surgical Pathology Report on Hysterectomies for Endometrial Cancer

- What procedure was performed, and what structures/organs are present?
- What is the size of the tumor?
- What are the histologic type and grade of neoplasm present?
- What is the maximum depth of tumor invasion (in millimeters)? (Measure from the normal endometrial/myometrial junction.)
- What is the total myometrial thickness at the deepest point of invasion (in millimeters)?
- What is the distance from the deepest tumor/myometrial junction to the serosa (in millimeters)?
- Does the tumor extend through the serosa?
- Does the tumor involve the endocervix? (Specify surface glandular and/or stromal involvement.)
- Is capillary–lymphatic space invasion seen?
- Does the tumor involve the adjacent adnexa?
- Does the tumor involve any lymph nodes? (Include the number of nodes involved and the number of nodes examined at each specified site.)

Radical Hysterectomy for Cervical Cancer

Radical hysterectomies are performed for early stage invasive squamous carcinomas and adenocarcinomas of the cervix. In addition to the uterus and cervix, the specimen has attached paracervical soft tissue and a vaginal cuff.

Begin by orienting, measuring, and weighing the uterus and cervix as described in the section on hysterectomies for benign disease. Also, measure the size of the attached paracervical tissue and the length of the attached vaginal cuff. Note whether the shape of the cervix is rounded or barrel shaped. Ink the right and left paracervical tissues, the anterior/posterior soft tissue margins of the cervical canal, and the vaginal cuff margin. Remove the paracervical tissue by shaving each side close to its lateral attachment on the cervix. Section this tissue at 0.3-cm inter-

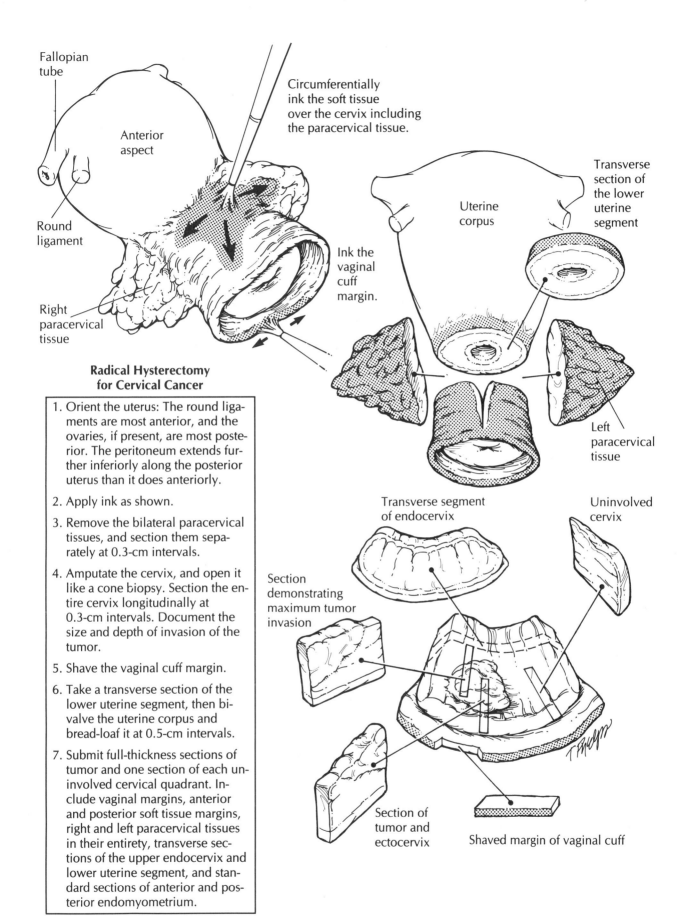

Fallopian tube

Anterior aspect

Round ligament

Right paracervical tissue

Circumferentially ink the soft tissue over the cervix including the paracervical tissue.

Ink the vaginal cuff margin.

Uterine corpus

Transverse section of the lower uterine segment

Left paracervical tissue

Transverse segment of endocervix

Uninvolved cervix

Section demonstrating maximum tumor invasion

Section of tumor and ectocervix

Shaved margin of vaginal cuff

Radical Hysterectomy for Cervical Cancer

1. Orient the uterus: The round ligaments are most anterior, and the ovaries, if present, are most posterior. The peritoneum extends further inferiorly along the posterior uterus than it does anteriorly.

2. Apply ink as shown.

3. Remove the bilateral paracervical tissues, and section them separately at 0.3-cm intervals.

4. Amputate the cervix, and open it like a cone biopsy. Section the entire cervix longitudinally at 0.3-cm intervals. Document the size and depth of invasion of the tumor.

5. Shave the vaginal cuff margin.

6. Take a transverse section of the lower uterine segment, then bivalve the uterine corpus and bread-loaf it at 0.5-cm intervals.

7. Submit full-thickness sections of tumor and one section of each uninvolved cervical quadrant. Include vaginal margins, anterior and posterior soft tissue margins, right and left paracervical tissues in their entirety, transverse sections of the upper endocervix and lower uterine segment, and standard sections of anterior and posterior endomyometrium.

vals, and submit the entire tissue for histologic examination. Any identifiable lymph nodes may be dissected and separately designated.

Next, amputate the cervix at the level of the internal os, and open the canal with a longitudinal incision opposite the tumor. Pin it open, and fix it as you would a cone biopsy. Measure the maximum tumor width and length as well as the distance to the nearest vaginal margin. Examine the vaginal cuff. Unless the tumor is close to the vaginal margin, the margin may be removed with a 0.3-cm parallel shave and submitted as four designated quadrants. If the tumor closely approaches the vaginal margin, leave the vaginal cuff intact and take perpendicular margins to demonstrate the relationship of the tumor to the margin. Serially section the cervix at 0.3-cm intervals, and measure the maximum tumor thickness as well as the thickness of the cervical wall at that site. Occasionally, a cervical tumor may not be easily discernible as a result of prior surgery or therapy.

Now turn your attention to the uterine corpus. Take a transverse section of the lower uterine segment and bivalve the uterus into anterior and posterior halves. Examine the corpus with serial transverse sections as you would in any hysterectomy specimen.

Sections for microscopic analysis should be chosen to demonstrate the maximum thickness of the tumor and its interface with any normal-appearing mucosa. If the tumor is not visible, the cervix with attached vaginal cuff should be entirely submitted as in a cone biopsy. The superior extent of the tumor can be documented by taking transverse sections of the upper endocervix and lower uterine segment. The inferior extent of the tumor is documented by taking sections of the cervical tumor that include the adjacent vaginal tissue. Margins to be evaluated include the left and right paracervical tissues, submitted in their entirety, and the vaginal cuff. The anterior and posterior cervical soft tissue margins should be submitted to delineate the extent of the tumor in relationship to the bladder and rectum.

Lymph nodes are usually submitted separately by the surgeon from the right and left internal iliac, external iliac, obturator, pelvic, and para-aortic node groups. They can be handled in a routine manner for evaluation of metastatic disease.

Important Issues to Address in Your Surgical Pathology Report on Radical Hysterectomies for Cervical Cancer

- What procedure was performed, and what structures/organs are present?
- What are the histologic type and grade of the tumor?
- Are any associated precursor lesions present (cervical intraepithelial neoplasia (CIN) or adenocarcinoma in situ (AIS))?
- What is the tumor size? (What is the maximum linear extent of invasion?)
- What is the maximum depth of invasion (in millimeters)? Measure from the base of the normal surface epithelium.
- What is the thickness of the cervical wall at the point of deepest tumor invasion (in millimeters)?
- Is the tumor unifocal or multifocal?
- Does the tumor involve capillary–lymphatic spaces?
- Does the tumor extend into the vagina, paracervical/parametrial tissue, or uterus?
- Does the tumor involve any resection margins?
- Is metastatic disease present? Record the number of lymph nodes with metastases and the number of lymph nodes identified by site.

Pelvic Exenterations Including Vaginectomies

Vaginectomies for vaginal cancer include a portion of vagina attached to the uterus and cervix. These specimens can be handled in the same manner as radical hysterectomies for cervical cancer, although the paracervical soft tissues may not be present. Important observations include the size of the tumor and the distance of the tumor to the vaginal margin. Sections should be taken so as to demonstrate the greatest depth of tumor invasion, the tumor with adjacent normal-appearing mucosa, and the relationship of the tumor to the cervix. If the bladder is included with the uterus the resection is termed an *anterior exenteration*, and if the rectum is included, the resection is termed a *post-*

Paracervical soft tissue

Uterus

Ureter

Bladder

Rectum

Urethra

Vagina

Proximal bowel margin

Total Pelvic Exenteration

1. Identify and measure each of the organs present.

2. Shave the vaginal, ureteral, and urethral margins, and inflate the bladder with formalin.

3. Fill the vagina with formalin-soaked gauze sponges.

4. Take perpendicular sections of the proximal and distal rectal margins, and inflate the rectum with formalin.

5. After fixation, bisect through the center of the specimen to divide it into right and left halves.

6. Identify and sample any lymph nodes in the paracervical soft tissue.

7. Submit sections of the cervical tumor and its relationship to the paracervical soft tissue, vagina, bladder, and rectum; standard endomyometrial, ovary, and fallopian tube sections; all lymph nodes and all margins to include bilateral ureters, urethra, vagina, and proximal and distal rectum.

Section of endomyometrium

Paracervical lymph node

Ureteral margin

Section demonstrating tumor invading bowel wall

Section demonstrating tumor invading bladder wall

Section demonstrating tumor involving proximal vagina

Distal bowel margin

Urethral margin

Vaginal margin

127

erior exenteration. With these added structures, additional sections include documentation of the extent of tumor involvement of the bladder or rectal wall, and an evaluation of their respective surgical margins. Specifically, these include the urethral and ureteral margins for the bladder, and the proximal and distal bowel margins for the rectum.

Exenterations are also performed for centrally recurrent cervical cancer. Perhaps the most daunting specimen received in the surgical pathology laboratory is a total pelvic exenteration, which includes the bladder, uterus with attached adnexa, vagina and rectum. The evaluation of these specimens uses both a separate and an integrated approach, as described in Chapter 6. Resection margins are best handled if each of the four main components (i.e., bladder, vagina, uterus, and rectum) is thought of separately. Appropriate examination of the central tumor involves demonstrating its *in situ* relationship to these surrounding organs.

When a total pelvic exenteration specimen is received for recurrent cervical cancer, do not panic. Instead, calmly note the organs present and their dimensions. Specifically, look for the ureters, urethra, bladder, uterus, fallopian tubes, ovaries, vagina, and rectum. Take shave sections of the vaginal, ureteral, and urethral margins. Take perpendicular sections from the proximal and distal rectal margins, providing ink for margin orientation. Next, ink all the exposed soft tissue that surrounds the cervix and tumor.

Fill the vagina with formalin-soaked gauze pads, and distend the bladder and rectum with formalin. Submerge the entire specimen in formalin, and fix it overnight. The fixed specimen may then be bisected in a sagittal plane to dem-

onstrate the tumor and its relationship to surrounding structures. This is best accomplished by using probes in the urethra and uterine canal as midline guides. After the specimen has been sectioned, a diagram can facilitate the description of the tumor, including its extension. Take sections of the tumor to demonstrate invasion of the bladder, rectum, vagina, and/or paracervical tissue. Document the vaginal and paracervical soft tissue margins with perpendicular or shave sections. Last, dissect the soft tissue surrounding the cervix, and submit for histology a section of any lymph nodes found.

Important Issues to Address in Your Surgical Pathology Report on Pelvic Exenterations

- What procedure was performed, and what structures/organs are present?
- What is the site of origin of the tumor?
- What are the histologic type and grade of the tumor?
- What is the size of the tumor?
- What other organs are involved by the tumor? Specify the extent of tumor involvement into these structures. That is, does it reach the muscular wall, submucosa, or mucosa?
- Does the tumor infiltrate the capillary–lymphatic spaces?
- Does the tumor involve any resection margins?
- Does the tumor involve any lymph nodes? (Include the number of nodes involved and the number of nodes examined at each specified site.)
- Are any radiation effects present?

24 Ovary and Fallopian Tube

Ovarian Biopsies and Wedge Resections

Biopsies and wedge resections of the ovary are infrequently performed procedures that are used primarily for the evaluation of infertility. Biopsies should be measured, briefly described as to color and texture, and submitted in their entirety. Wedge resections should also be weighed and evaluated for capsule thickening, "powder burns" of endometriosis, subcortical cysts, and yellow stromal nodularity indicating hyperthecosis. Sections should be taken perpendicular to the ovarian surface to demonstrate the relationship of the capsule, cortex, and medulla.

Salpingectomies

Fallopian tubes can be removed in part or in total. Partial salpingectomies are commonly performed for tubal sterilization. Total salpingectomies are performed for ectopic pregnancies, in conjunction with an oophorectomy, or as part of a hysterectomy specimen. Salpingectomies for primary neoplasms of the fallopian tube are uncommon.

The evaluation of the incidental salpingectomy specimen is straightforward. The gross appearance of the tube is usually unremarkable. Record the length, diameter, and color of the tube. Describe any features in relationship to the different portions of the fallopian tube. The intramural portion lies within the uterus and is not seen in separate salpingectomies. The isthmic portion is the first 2 to 3 cm external to the uterus. The ampullary portion is the next 5 to 8 cm, and the infundibulum starts where the tube begins to widen and encompasses the fimbriated end. The patency of the lumen may be tested with a blunt-tipped probe. Serially section the fallopian tube at 0.5-cm intervals, and examine it for nodularity, cysts, or masses. Submit one transverse section from each region.

Small segments of intervening fallopian tube are usually submitted in tubal sterilizaton procedures. For legal purposes, a *complete* cross section of each fallopian tube must be microscopically documented.

Salpingectomies for ectopic pregnancy should be examined for signs of rupture. Serially section the fallopian tube, and submit any tissue with the gross appearance of products of conception. Be sure to include the adjacent wall. If no products of conception are grossly identified, submit several sections from the wall in regions of hemorrhage as well as several from the intraluminal clot. In contrast to uterine products of conception, in which villi are seldom seen within the blood clots, villi are often identified in the clots from ectopic pregnancies. Sections of uninvolved fallopian tube should also be submitted to look for evidence of tubal disease contributing to the occurrence of an ectopic pregnancy (e.g., chronic salpingitis, endometriosis, or salpingitis isthmica nodosa).

A salpingectomy for tubal carcinoma should be evaluated in the same manner as an incidental salpingectomy. In addition, the size, location, and extent of the tumor should be documented. The maximum depth of tumor penetration can be evaluated with full-thickness transverse sections of the tube. Margins include the cut edge of the broad ligament and the proximal fallopian tube end, if not submitted with the uterus.

Ovarian Cystectomies and Oophorectomies

Ovarian cystectomies and oophorectomies are evaluated in a similar manner. Oophorectomies may be accompanied by the fallopian tube or may be part of a total hysterectomy specimen. A portion of broad ligament may also be present as the ovary attaches to the posterior surface of the broad ligament and lies inferior to the fallopian tube.

Incidental oophorectomies are easily handled. Record the weight and dimensions of the ovary. Examine the outer surface for cysts, nodules, or adhesions. Bivalve the ovary with a cut through its longest dimension and mid-hilum. Evaluate the sectioned surface for any cysts or nodules, and designate their location as either cortical, medullary, or hilar. Keep in mind that the appearance of the ovary will vary considerably with the age and the reproductive status of the woman. The normal ovary in the reproductive years can measure up to 4 cm, whereas an ovary this size in a postmenopausal woman warrants close evaluation.

Cystectomies are usually performed for benign lesions or in women with ovarian masses who wish to preserve their fertility. The most common indication is for the removal of a dermoid cyst. After weighing and measuring the cyst, examine the external surface for evidence of rupture. Place the cyst in a container, and carefully make a small incision in the wall to allow its contents to be drained. Note the color and consistency of the cyst fluid. Continue the incision with a pair of scissors to expose the entire inner surface. The thick sebaceous fluid within a dermoid cyst may have to be removed by rinsing briefly with hot water. Examine the cyst lining, and look for any regions of granularity or papillary projections. In dermoid cysts, look for Rokitansky's tubercle, which appears as a firm, nodular excrescence. This region and any other thickened areas should be submitted in their entirety to look for evidence of immature elements. Large, unilocular cysts with a smooth inner lining may be cut in strips and submitted like placental membrane rolls to get a maximum view of the cyst wall. Cystectomies for lesions other than unilocular smooth-walled cysts or dermoid cysts should be handled as described next.

Oophorectomies for ovarian tumors can be quite large and heavy. Often, the only recognizable structure is the fallopian tube, which may be attenuated and stretched over the ovarian surface. Begin by weighing and measuring the specimen. Closely examine the surface for evidence of rupture, adhesions, or nodular tumor excrescences. Ink these regions for orientation. Section the ovarian mass at 1-cm intervals through its longest axis. If the mass is cystic, you may want to perform this in a pan or on a work station that allows for easy drainage of fluid. Remember to document the color and consistency of the cyst fluid. Is the fluid serous, mucinous, or hemorrhagic? Note whether the mass is solid, cystic, or both. If both, document the percentage of each region. Examine the surfaces of the cysts for evidence of granularity, nodules, or papillary projections. The thickness of the cyst walls should also be recorded. Describe any regions of hemorrhage or necrosis. Try to find any residual ovarian parenchyma. This is commonly found in the region immediately adjacent to the fallopian tube. If a stromal or steroid cell tumor is suspected, tissue should be saved frozen in case fat stains are needed. Fresh tumor should also be saved frozen for possible estrogen/progesterone receptor assays. Photographs of the cut surface can aid in documentation of the mass and for designating where sections were taken. At this point, it may be helpful to fix the 1-cm slices in formalin before further manipulation.

Historically, ovarian tumors are submitted with a minimum of one section per 1 to 2 cm of the greatest tumor dimension. This rule is especially useful in the case of mucinous tumors, which tend to have only focal regions demonstrating atypical or frankly invasive elements. If the tumor is uniform throughout, as many serous tumors are, fewer sections may be prudent. In general, sections should be submitted from regions that are solid, hemorrhagic, or necrotic. Cysts that show granular, nodular, or papillary excrescences should be thoroughly sampled. Also include any regions that appear sieve-like or honeycombed. Multiple large unilocular cysts may be more judi-

Regions of the fallopian tube

Isthmus Ampulla Infundibulum

Fimbriae

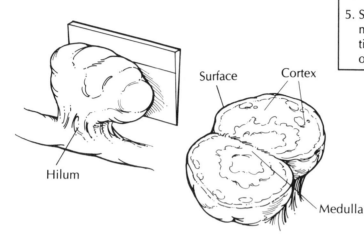

Hilum

Surface Cortex

Medulla

Incidental Salpingo-oophorectomy

1. Identify the fimbriated end of the fallopian tube. Record the length and diameter of the tube.

2. Probe the lumen for patency.

3. Serially section the fallopian tube at 0.5-cm intervals. Submit one transverse section from each of the isthmic, ampullary, and infundibular regions.

4. Weigh and measure the ovary.

5. Section the ovary through its longest dimension and hilum. Submit one section for every 2 cm of non-neoplastic ovary.

Salpingo-oophorectomy for an Ovarian Mass

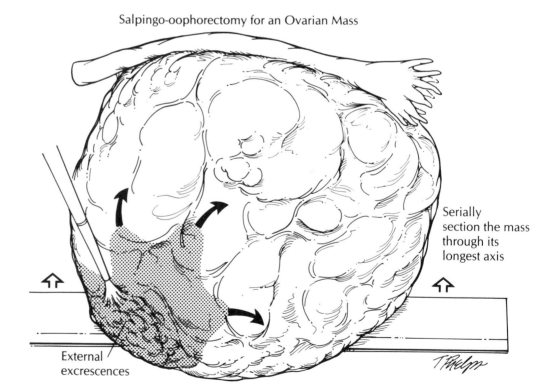

Serially section the mass through its longest axis

External excrescences

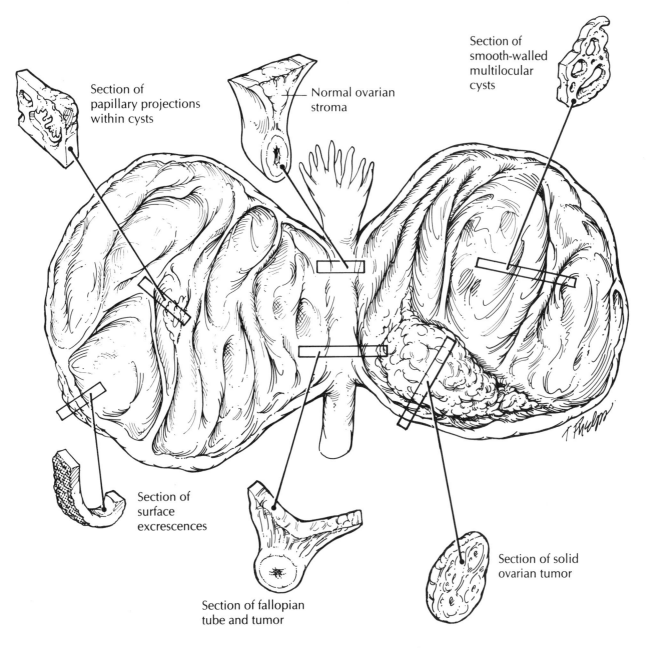

Section of papillary projections within cysts

Normal ovarian stroma

Section of smooth-walled multilocular cysts

Section of surface excrescences

Section of fallopian tube and tumor

Section of solid ovarian tumor

Salpingo-oophorectomy for an Ovarian Mass

1. Weigh and measure the mass. Identify the fallopian tube, if present.

2. Carefully inspect the ovarian surface for evidence of rupture, adhesions, or tumor excrescences.

3. Ink any external surface excrescences, and section the ovarian mass at 1- to 2-cm intervals through its longest axis. If the mass is cystic, note the color and consistency of the cyst contents.

4. Submit one section per 1 to 2 cm of tumor diameter. Direct sampling to emphasize solid, papillary, necrotic, and hemorrhagic regions. Include any surface excrescences, extension to the fallopian tube, and any residual ovary.

ciously sampled. Sections that demonstrate the junction between the ovary and adjacent fallopian tube, as well as any residual ovary, should also be submitted.

Specimens for Ovarian Tumor Staging

The staging procedure for an ovarian tumor can include an omentectomy, multiple biopsies of the peritoneum, and lymph node dissections.

Omentectomy specimens should be weighed, measured, and serially sectioned at 0.5-cm intervals to look for gross tumor nodules. Palpate the fat for areas of induration or small miliary nodules. For grossly visible tumor involvement, one to three representative sections should be submitted for histology. If the tumor is not grossly visible, take multiple sections from the firmest regions in the omental fat.

Peritoneal small biopsies should be routinely processed and submitted in their entirety. If the tumor extensively involves the pelvic peritoneum, a cavitronic ultrasonic surgical aspirator may be used to remove the implants. Tissue removed this way can be handled like a curettage specimen.

Lymph nodes are received separately and designated by location. They can be handled in a routine manner for evaluation of metastatic disease.

Important Issues to Address in Your Surgical Pathology Report on Ovarian Tumors

- What procedure was performed, and what structures/organs are present?
- Is a neoplasm present? Is it of epithelial, sex-cord/stromal, germ cell, or metastatic origin?
- What are the size, histologic type, and grade of the neoplasm?
- Was the ovarian capsule ruptured?
- Does the tumor involve the ovarian capsule?
- Does the tumor involve the adjacent fallopian tube or broad ligament?
- If submitted, does the tumor involve the contralateral ovary and/or the serosa or parenchyma of the uterus?
- Does the tumor involve the omentum?
- Does the tumor involve any lymph nodes? (Include the number of nodes involved and the number of nodes examined at each specified site.)
- Do the soft tissue staging biopsies show tumor implants? If so, specify whether they are invasive or noninvasive.

25 Products of Conception and Placentas

Products of Conception

Products of conception is the term used for intra-uterine tissue that is either passed spontaneously or removed surgically in early gestation. These specimens are usually sent for diagnostic or therapeutic purposes. The major goal is to verify that a gestation was present. This requires the identification of either fetal parts, chorionic villi, or trophoblastic cells. The presence of decidua alone is not suffecient for diagnosis. Molar pregnancies and placental neoplasia may also be identified, although these are much less common. Always be familiar with the patient's clinical history, as this will help guide your examination.

Specimens from first trimester gestations are usually composed of irregularly shaped small tissue fragments and blood clots suspended within a fluid-filled container. Strain the entire contents of the container, and give an estimate of the amount of the specimen by volume (in cubic centimeters) or as an aggregate measurement. Spread the specimen across your work bench, and separate the blood clots from the tissue. Carefully inspect the tissue for fetal parts and villous tissue. Villous tissue is soft and spongy, whereas decidua is more likely to be firmer and membranous. Another method of examination is to suspend the tissue fragments in saline. The delicate villous fronds will then become readily apparent. Also, look for evidence of swollen or hydropic villi, which appear as small, grape-like vesicles.

If fetal parts are identified, measure them separately, and submit several pieces along with representative villous tissue in one or two tissue cassettes. If no fetal parts are identified and you are confident of your identification of villi, submit representative sections in two to three tissue cassettes. However, because the confirmation of an intrauterine pregnancy is often needed immediately, it may be wise to use the following guideline: Submit the entire specimen if it is small or submit as much as can be included in five tissue cassettes. Always specify the percentage of the specimen that was submitted, and include only tissue fragments. We have found that the microscopic evaluation of blood clots from intrauterine pregnancies often does not reveal entrapped villi. If no villi are identified after your initial microscopic evaluation, the entire specimen may need to be submitted.

In the case of a clinically suspected molar pregnancy or the presence of hydropic villi, the submission of at least eight tissue cassettes is recommended to assess the degree of trophoblast proliferation. Any large tissue fragments, that is, fragments greater than 3 to 4 cm, should be sectioned and entirely submitted if they are firm, indurated, or necrotic.

Second trimester therapeutic or elective abortion specimens may have intact placentas and fetuses. These specimens may be handled in the routine surgical pathology laboratory if the fetus is less than 500 g and/or less than 20 to 21 weeks' gestation. A description of a full neonatal autopsy is beyond the scope of this chapter; however, most cases can be appropriately handled with a limited approach. Briefly, weigh the fetus, and measure the crown–rump, crown–heel, and foot length. Examine the external appearance for skin slippage and any gross abnormalities of structure such as missing limbs or extra digits. Open the thorax and abdomen with a vertical midline incision. Confirm the appropriate position of the internal organs, and take a piece of liver, lung, and gonads for microscopic evaluation. For the examination of a fetus with either chromosomal or congenital abnormalities, the reader is referred to Wigglesworth.[4] The placenta can be routinely handled, as described in the next section.

Placentas

Placentas are submitted for evaluation because of maternal conditions, fetal/neonatal conditions, gross anomalies of the placenta, and in all multiple gestations. Many abnormalities can be recognized with a thorough gross examination. Approach each placenta by systematically evaluating the three main components: the fetal membranes, the umbilical cord, and the placental disc.

Placentas should initially be examined in the fresh, unfixed state. Choose a work area that allows for the drainage of blood and fluid, which is copiously expressed from the placental bed on sectioning. Always be aware of the clinical history before proceeding, and check the contents of the container that the placenta was received in for any separate blood clots. Orient the placenta by placing the spongy, red maternal surface face down and the shiny, membranous fetal surface with umbilical cord face up. Invert the membranes, if necessary, so that they are draped around the fetal surface.

Begin your examination with the fetal membranes, noting their color, lucency, and insertion. Normal membranes should be shiny and clear and should insert at the edge of the placental disc. Look for any opacities, which may indicate inflammation; small white nodules, which indicate amnion nodosum; and meconium staining, which may indicate intrauterine fetal hypoxia. As illustrated, membrane insertion within the circumference of the fetal surface is called *placenta extrachorialis* and can be subdivided into either circummarginate (a smooth chorionic surface at the insertion), or circumvallate (a grooved or ridged chorionic surface at the insertion). Both may reflect previous bleeding from earlier placental separation. Next, re-create the gestational sac by gently lifting the membranes, and cut a 2- to 3-cm-wide strip of membrane

from the ruptured margin to the placental margin. Beginning at the ruptured end, roll the membrane strip with the amnion inward around a small probe. Remove the probe, and cut the newly created "membrane roll" transversely for histologic examination. The membranes can now be removed by trimming them along the placental margin.

The umbilical cord is examined next. Record its length and site of insertion. Although the length provided may be artificially shortened if a segment was removed in the delivery room, excessively short (less than 30 cm) or long (more than 70 cm) cords are significant because of their association with abnormal fetal development and activity. Insertions at the edge of the placenta or in the membranes may be associated with exposed vessels, which should be examined carefully for any tears or thrombi. Remove the umbilical cord at its insertion, and examine the entire length of the cord for thinning, thrombi, or knots. True knots can be undone when the umbilical cord ends are freed, whereas false knots cannot. Make several transverse cuts along the cord, and examine the vessels. There should be two small thick-walled arteries and one large thin-walled vein. At the insertion site, many vessels join together and they may not be fused into their terminal vessel until just above this point. Also, twisted regions of the umbilical cord can give the artificial appearance of an increased number of vessels on cross section. Therefore, for an accurate documentation of the number of vessels, it is best to submit a transverse section of the umbilical cord for examination from an area that is not excessively twisted and at least 1 cm above the insertion site.

The placenta should now be a solitary disk. Record its weight and three-dimensional measurement. Any unusual shapes or extra lobes should be noted. Examine the membranes on the fetal surface first, and look for nodules within or just below the amnion/chorion layer. Superficial white nodules or fine granularity may represent amnion nodosum, whereas firm, yellowish nodules beneath the membranes may represent subchorionic fibrin deposition. If present, these should be sampled for histology. Next, examine the vessels that radiate toward the umbilical cord, and look for tears or thrombi. Turn the placenta over, and examine the maternal surface. The cotyledons should be relatively uniform and intact. Look for any evidence

Roll the membrane strip around a probe with the amnion inward.

Section transversely to create a "jelly roll."

Umbilical cord

Placental disk

Fetal surface

Artery

Vein

Villous parenchyma

Maternal surface

Full-thickness section of the placental disk

Fetal half

Maternal half

Single and Twin Placentas

1. Orient the placenta with the maternal surface down and the membranes up, encircling the fetal surface.

2. Open the gestational sac, and cut a 2- to 3-cm strip of membrane from the ruptured margin to the placental margin. Roll this strip along a probe with the amnion inward, and section it transversely.

3. Note the insertion of the membranes and trim the membranes from the placental disk.

4. Measure the umbilical cord, remove it at its insertion, and make several transverse sections along its length. Note the number of vessels.

5. Weigh and measure the placental disk.

6. Section the parenchyma at 1- to 2-cm intervals with the maternal surface upward.

7. Submit two to three full-thickness sections of the placental disk. These may be divided into fetal and maternal halves. Also, submit membrane roll and umbilical cord cross sections. For multiple gestations, include the dividing membrane and T zone.

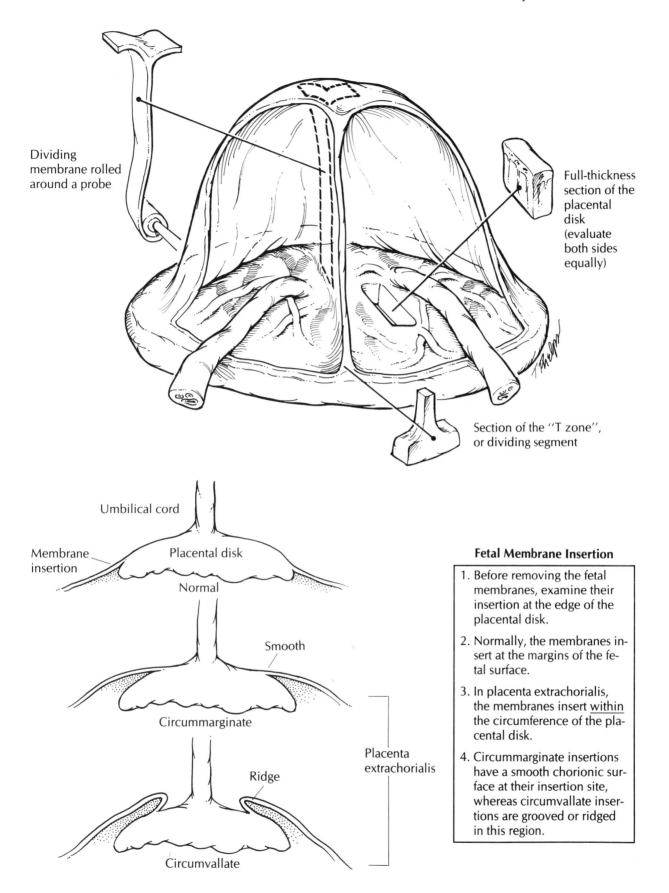

Dividing membrane rolled around a probe

Full-thickness section of the placental disk (evaluate both sides equally)

Section of the "T zone", or dividing segment

Umbilical cord

Placental disk

Membrane insertion

Normal

Smooth

Circummarginate

Ridge

Placenta extrachorialis

Circumvallate

Fetal Membrane Insertion

1. Before removing the fetal membranes, examine their insertion at the edge of the placental disk.

2. Normally, the membranes insert at the margins of the fetal surface.

3. In placenta extrachorialis, the membranes insert <u>within</u> the circumference of the placental disk.

4. Circummarginate insertions have a smooth chorionic surface at their insertion site, whereas circumvallate insertions are grooved or ridged in this region.

of disruption or indentation of the parenchyma. Adherent clots without underlying compression do not necessarily signify a placental abruption. Serially section the placenta at 1- to 2-cm intervals with the maternal surface upward, and examine the parenchyma. The greatest thickness of the placenta from the fetal to the maternal surface should be measured. Look for infarcts, intervillous thrombi, or tumors. Both infarcts and intervillous thrombi can appear yellow or white. Intervillous thrombi are usually smooth and displace the villous parenchyma, whereas infarcts involve the villous tissue and appear more granular. If an infarct is identified, be sure to specify the percentage of parenchyma that is involved. Tumors are rare in the placenta, but hemangiomas, choriocarcinomas, and metastatic cancers can be found.

Sections should be taken to include the full thickness of the placenta from the central regions, rather than from the margins. If the section is too thick to fit into one tissue cassette, it may be divided into maternal and fetal halves. Standard sections include two central sections from different cotyledons and any focal lesions.

Fused placentas from multiple gestations can be evaluated in a similar manner to single gestations. Additional handling includes an examination of the dividing membranes and the identification of any vascular anastomoses. Dividing membranes are composed of two outer amnions and either one or two intervening chorions. All monochorionic placentas come from monozygotic (identical) twins, whereas dichorionic placentas may belong to either monozygotic or dizygotic (fraternal) twins. The dividing membrane can be easily peeled apart in monochorionic placentas. Dichorionic placentas are more opaque and difficult to separate. Although you can perform this separation yourself, histologic verification is necessary, and a membrane roll should be submitted from a region that has not been separated. A section from the "T zone," where the membranes attach to the fetal surface, may also be submitted. Look for any vascular anastomoses between the two sides. Note whether these are artery-to-artery (AA), vein-to-vein (VV), or artery-to-vein (AV). Arteries can be readily recognized by the fact that they lie on top of the veins. Abnormal anastomoses may be reflected by one side being severely congested and large, with the other being pale and small.

Additional Studies

You may be requested to send cultures or cytogenetic studies on obstetric specimens. For aerobic and anaerobic cultures of the placenta, it is best to sear a small region of the membranes over the placental disk with a heated scalpel and then sample the underlying subchorionic zone. This technique reduces surface contamination. For cytogenetic studies, small fragments of villous tissue, skin, or pericardium from a fetus can be submitted in sterile media containers provided by the cytogenetics laboratory. It is best to remove this tissue with clean, but not necessarily sterile, instruments. Avoid areas with obvious bacterial contamination.

Important Issues to Address in Your Surgical Pathology Report on Placentas

- What procedure was performed (was the placenta removed via spontaneous delivery or manually), and what structures/organs are present?
- What is the trimester maturation of the villi (second or third trimester)?
- Are any abnormalities of the placental shape, membrane insertion, or cord insertion present?
- Are any anomalous vessels or vessels with thrombi present?
- Is a normal three-vessel cord present?
- Is there inflammation of the membranes, umbilical cord, or chorionic villi?
- Are the maternal cotyledons disrupted or is there compression by hematomas?
- Does the parenchyma show any infarction? If so, what percentage is involved?
- Are any villous thrombi or neoplasms identified in the parenchyma?
- In twin gestations, is a dividing membrane present? If so, is it monochorionic–diamniotic or dichorionic–diamniotic?

VIII   The Urinary Tract and Male Genital System

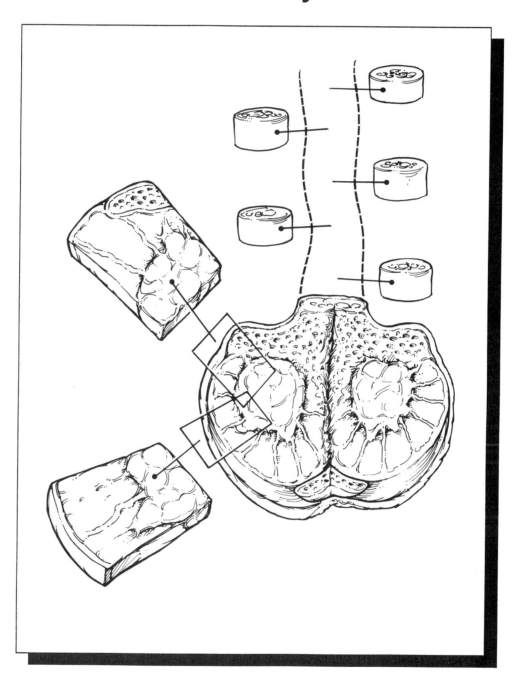

26 Penis

Foreskin

Foreskins removed from infants are usually not submitted to the surgical pathology laboratory for examination. If you do receive one of these specimens, measure it, describe its appearance, and submit a section for histologic evaluation. Foreskins removed from older patients are routinely submitted for evaluation, because they are more likely to harbor pathology. You need to sample these specimens more extensively and pay close attention to the margin of resection. Ink the epithelial margin, and carefully inspect the surfaces of the specimen. Record the number, size, location, and appearance of any lesions. Because the foreskin is much easier to section once it is fixed, pin the four corners of the foreskin onto a wax tablet, and submerge the specimen in formalin.

Even if no lesions are appreciated on gross inspection, liberally sample foreskins removed from adults to look for early neoplastic changes. Use perpendicular sections so that the epithelial margin is included in the sections. When a neoplasm is suspected, each quadrant of the epithelial margin should be sampled. More extensive sampling may be necessary if a visible lesion is large or if the lesion approaches the margin at several sites.

Penectomies

The diverse findings encountered in penectomies range from the essentially normal penis removed from a patient undergoing a sex change operation, to the penis grossly distorted by gangrene or infiltrating carcinoma. The best way to be prepared for virtually any penectomy specimen is to become familiar with the anatomy of the normal penis. This familiarity will allow you to answer those questions that should be foremost in mind when evaluating a penile lesion: Where on the penis does the lesion arise, into what anatomic compartments does the lesion extend, and how close is it to the resection margin?

Before beginning the dissection, identify the three basic structural components of the penis as illustrated. The *shaft*, as its name suggests, is the cylindrical rod-like portion of the penis. It is covered by a loosely attached layer of rugated skin, and it houses the three erectile bodies of the penis—the two corpora cavernosa (located dorsally and laterally) and the single corpus spongiosum (located ventrally, surrounding the urethra along the midline). The *glans* is the conical-shaped expansion of the distal corpus spongiosum. It sits like a bonnet on the end of the shaft. The edge of the glans at its base is referred to as the corona, and at the apex of the glans is the opening of the urethra (i.e., the urethral meatus). The *foreskin* is a retractable fold of skin that partially covers the glans. Its attachment to the skin of the shaft occurs just behind the corona. The foreskin will obviously not be present in penectomies from circumcised males.

Carefully examine the surfaces of the specimen, keeping in mind that the vast majority of penile neoplasms arise from the surface epithelium of the glans and from the undersurface of the foreskin. Some neoplasms may be concealed by the foreskin, so be sure to retract this

Glans

Corona

Shaft

Corpora cavernosa

Turn the penis over and open the urethra.

Corpus spongiosum

Urethra

Bisect the penis using the opened urethra as a guide.

Longitudinal section through the glans

T Phelps.

Penectomy

1. Identify the shaft and the glans. Remove the foreskin (if present), along the corona.

2. Take a complete shave section of the amputation margin, and bread-loaf the shaft of the penis as shown.

3. Open the urethra with scissors, then use the urethra as a guide to bisect the glans longitudinally.

4. Document the size and depth of invasion of any neoplasms.

5. Submit sections of tumor, foreskin, transverse sections through the shaft, and longitudinal sections through the glans. Submit the amputation margin as a shave section.

skin fold, and look at the entire surface including the epithelium lining the deep recesses of the coronal sulcus. Other neoplasms—especially those that are not deeply invasive—may be so subtle as to elude casual inspection; therefore, be sure to look carefully for discolored plaque-like irregularities that characterize superficial spreading carcinomas. Do not stop once one lesion has been found, but keep looking for others. Squamous carcinomas of the penis tend to be multifocal, and these tumors will be overlooked if the entire epithelial surface is not examined.

In the gross description, record the dimensions of the entire specimen and the dimensions of each of its individual components (i.e., foreskin, glans, and shaft). Describe the surfaces of each component, and note the number, size, color, and distribution of any lesions found. Assess the tumor's macroscopic pattern of growth (e.g., nodular, ulcerative/infiltrative, verrucous, or flat).

Begin the dissection by taking a shave section from the penile shaft at the amputation site. This section represents the only margin. If it is carefully taken, this section will include margins of the skin, erectile bodies, and penile urethra. If all of these components cannot be included in a single section, submit each component individually. Remove the foreskin from the uncircumcised penectomy. This can be done with a circular cut leaving a 5-mm rim of foreskin attached to the corona. The foreskin should then be separately processed according to the guidelines given previously in the section on the foreskin. The deep structures of the penis are most easily visualized when the penis is sectioned in two different planes. Bread-loaf the shaft perpendicular to its long axis. Begin at the proximal end of the specimen, and stop 1 to 2 cm from the corona. Next, serially section the distal penis parallel to its long axis. The first of these parallel sections along the long axis should bisect the proximal penis into equal halves midline through the urethra. This is not a difficult section if you first use scissors to open the urethra at the 6-o'clock position (i.e., mid-ventral plane), and then insert a knife into the opened urethra to complete the longitudinal section. Serially section the rest of the glans parallel to this initial cut in the sagittal plane.

Examine the cut surfaces of the specimen. Locate and describe the appearance of the penile urethra, the corpus spongiosum, and the corpora cavernosa. If a tumor is present, measure how deeply it infiltrates the penis, and try to determine which anatomic structures the tumor involves. The standard sections that should be submitted for histologic evaluation include the following: (1) a shave section from the shaft margin (including the skin, erectile bodies, and urethra); (2) sections of foreskin; (3) transverse sections through the shaft at two or three different levels; and (4) longitudinal sections through the glans including a midline section with the urethra. When sampling the tumor, submit sections that demonstrate its relationships to the adjacent surface epithelium, to the urethra, and to the erectile bodies. For tumors that involve the urethra, determine the maximum tumor extension by submitting sections at regular intervals along the entire length of the penis.

Important Issues to Address in Your Surgical Pathology Report on Penectomies

- What procedure was performed, and what structures/organs are present?
- Is a neoplasm present?
- Where is the tumor located (e.g., foreskin, glans, shaft, and/or urethra)?
- Is the tumor *in situ* or infiltrating?
- What are the histologic type and grade of the tumor?
- What is the size of the tumor, and how deeply (in millimeters) does the tumor infiltrate the penis?
- Is vascular invasion identified?
- What deep structures does the tumor involve (e.g., subepithelial connective tissues, corpus spongiosum, corpora cavernosa, urethra, prostate, adjacent structures)?
- Are the resection margins free of tumor?
- Does the non-neoplastic portion of the penis show any pathology?

27 Prostate

Biopsies

Needle biopsies of the prostate consist of delicate and thin cores of tan soft tissue. Measure each piece of tissue, and document the total number of pieces before carefully transferring them into a tissue cassette. As is true for any small biopsy, do not use forceps to pick up these biopsies, because forceps can squeeze and distort the tissue. Have the histology laboratory section these biopsies at multiple levels, then have them stain alternating levels for routine histology. If sections are later needed for additional studies (e.g., immunoperoxidase), the unstained slides will be readily available, and diagnostic material will not be lost during sectioning of the tissue block.

Transurethral Resections and Open Enucleations

Frequently, the central region of the prostate is removed—either by transurethral resection or by open enucleation—to relieve symptoms of urinary obstruction caused by nodules compressing the prostatic urethra. Although the majority of these nodules are entirely benign, a small, yet significant percentage (i.e., 10%) harbor a carcinoma.

Tissue fragments obtained from transurethral resections of the prostate—referred to as *prostate chips*—are generally tan, rubbery, and cylindrical. The total number of chips resected varies greatly from case to case. Measure the combined weight of the chips, and record their aggregate dimensions. For larger specimens, it is not practical to submit all of the chips for histologic evaluation. Although six to eight tissue cassettes are generally sufficient to detect the vast majority of incidental carcinomas, the sensitivity of sampling can be increased by selectively submitting those chips that appear yellow, indurated, or in any other way grossly suspicious for carcinoma. More extensive sampling is warranted in specimens from younger patients, since even a small focus of carcinoma in these men may require aggressive therapy. For patients under the age of 65, consider submitting the entire specimen for histologic evaluation. Similarly, if cancer is identified histologically in a specimen that was partially submitted, the entire specimen should be submitted so that the approximate volume of the cancer can be calculated.

Specimens obtained by open enucleation are either partially or totally intact nodules, but the anatomic orientation of these nodules is usually not practical or possible. After weighing and measuring the tissue, serially section the specimen at 2- to 3-mm intervals. Note the appearance of the cut surface. Again, extensively sample the specimen to detect incidental carcinomas. Submit up to six to eight cassettes of tissue. As was true for the prostate chips, remember to selectively sample areas that appear grossly suspicious for carcinoma.

Radical Prostatectomies

One of the challenges of the dissection of radical prostatectomies is to find a balance which will maximize prognostic information while mini-

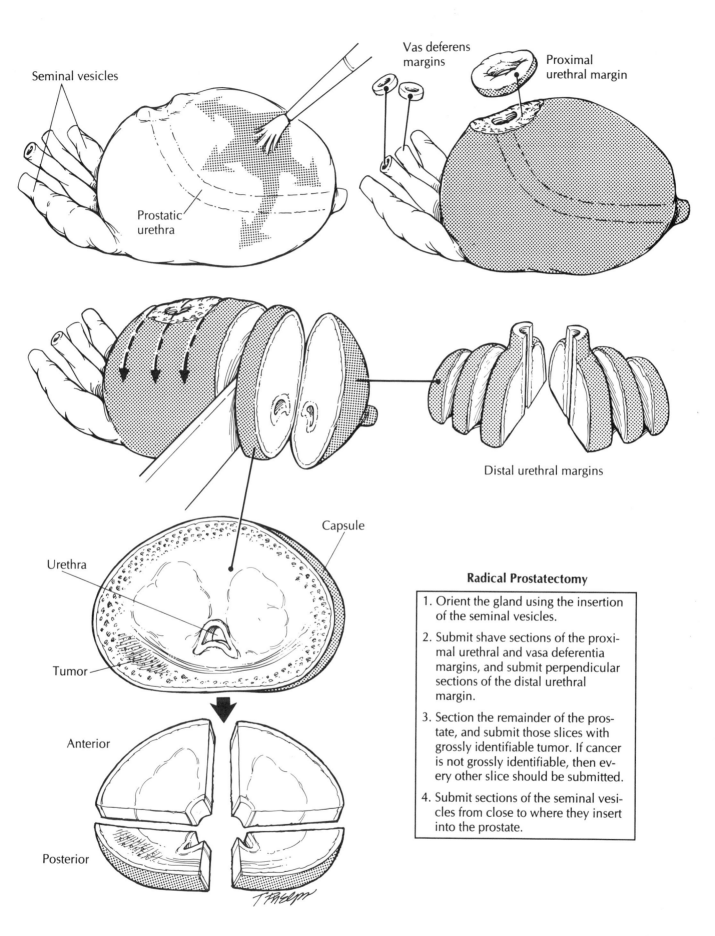

Seminal vesicles

Prostatic urethra

Vas deferens margins

Proximal urethral margin

Distal urethral margins

Capsule

Urethra

Tumor

Anterior

Posterior

Radical Prostatectomy

1. Orient the gland using the insertion of the seminal vesicles.

2. Submit shave sections of the proximal urethral and vasa deferentia margins, and submit perpendicular sections of the distal urethral margin.

3. Section the remainder of the prostate, and submit those slices with grossly identifiable tumor. If cancer is not grossly identifiable, then every other slice should be submitted.

4. Submit sections of the seminal vesicles from close to where they insert into the prostate.

mizing the number of tissue cassettes submitted. Selective sampling of a carcinoma of the prostate can be difficult because subtle differences in the gross appearance of cancer and non-neoplastic prostate tissue can be hard to recognize. This is why it is so important that you familiarize yourself with the subtleties of the gross appearance of prostate cancer. A number of the gross features of prostate cancer are outlined in Table 27-1, and these can be helpful in distinguishing carcinoma from non-neoplastic tissue.

Orient the prostate by locating the seminal vesicles and vasa deferentia. These structures insert into the posterior aspect of the base (proximal end) of the gland and provide a landmark that is quick and easy to find. In contrast to the broad and flat base, the apex (distal end) of the prostate narrows and becomes cone shaped. The contour of the gland can be used to distinguish the anterior and posterior aspects of the prostate. The anterior surface of the prostate is rounded and convex, while the posterior surface is broad and flat. After orienting the specimen, weigh and measure it. Inspect the intact prostate for asymmetry, and palpate it for areas of induration. Paint the surfaces of the prostate with ink, then fix the specimen in formalin for 18 to 24 hours.

Following fixation, thinly shave the vasa deferentia and the proximal urethral margins. The distal urethral margin can be submitted in one of two ways. One method is to submit this margin as a thinly shaved section. A second method is illustrated. Amputate the distal 1 cm of the apex, then section this apical cone at right angles to the cut edge in thin parallel slices. This latter technique allows for a more accurate assessment of exactly how close the cancer approaches the distal urethral margin. After the margins have been taken, serially section the prostate at 2- to 3-mm intervals from apex to base. Do not use the urethra as a point of reference for these sections, because this structure follows a curved course through the prostate. Instead, section the prostate perpendicular to the broad flat posterior surface of the gland. The carefully sectioned prostate can be likened to a loaf of sliced bread. Each individual slice should be intact, uniformly thin, and surrounded by a "crust" of prostatic capsule and inked soft tissue. You will come to realize the importance of this crust when you later have to evaluate the histologic sections for capsular penetration by the carcinoma and for the extension of the carcinoma to the soft tissue margin.

Lay the individual slices out sequentially from apex (distal) to base (proximal). Be careful to maintain the orientation (i.e., right vs. left, anterior vs. posterior) of each slice. Beginning at the apex and proceeding to the base, designate each slice (e.g., A, B, C, etc.). This will enable you to remember the location of each individual slice within the prostate.

Several key landmarks guide the examination of the individual slices. The prostatic urethra is located near the center of each slice. It has a roughly U-shaped appearance on cut section. The arms of the U point to the posterior surface of the gland, and its convexity points to the an-

---

TABLE 27-1. Gross appearance of prostate cancer.

Location: The cut surface of the normal prostate shows a fibromuscular band that divides the prostate into a peripheral zone and a transitional zone (i.e., periurethral area). Most carcinomas arise peripherally in the posterior and posterolateral portion of the gland. In contrast, hyperplastic nodules tend to be located centrally around the urethra.

Texture: Carcinomas tend to be solid and homogeneous, while non-neoplastic prostate tissue is often spongy and cystic.

Color: Carcinomas vary in color from gray to brown to yellow. Sometimes these colors contrast sharply with the uniform tan appearance of non-neoplastic prostate. Perhaps more commonly, the color of the cancer and non-neoplastic tissue overlap, and color cannot be used to distinguish the two.

Structural Alterations: Prostatic carcinomas often cause structural changes that are apparent on close inspection of the cut surface. Important clues to search for are asymmetry between the two sides of the gland and displacement of the fibromuscular band that normally divides the transitional and peripheral zones of the gland.

terior surface. Find the fibromuscular band of tissue that separates the central/anterior portion of the gland from the horseshoe-shaped peripheral portion of the gland. Try to find the cancer using the guidelines outlined in Table 27.1. Describe the appearance of any lesions, carefully noting their location (left or right, anterior or posterior) and size. Because each slice has already been designated, you can precisely indicate in your gross description which of the slices appear involved.

Finally, submit sections of each seminal vesicle. These should be taken close to where the seminal vesicles insert into the prostate. The number of sections of the prostate parenchyma that should be submitted depends on whether or not a carcinoma was identified on gross examination. If you can confidently identify the cancer, then submit those slices containing the entire gross lesion. If you cannot identify the cancer, then submit every other slice (e.g., A, C, E, etc.) of the prostate. The slices may have to be sectioned further to fit into standard tissue cassettes. A median section through the urethra will divide the slice into roughly equal right and left sides, and a coronal section through the urethra will, when necessary, further divide the slice into anterior and posterior quadrants. After the specimen has been appropriately sampled, retain the remaining tissue sections in their original order and orientation in case additional sections must be submitted. One simple method is to fasten the slices together with a safety pin or rubber band.

Pelvic Lymph Node Dissection

Radical prostatectomies are usually accompanied by a dissection of the pelvic lymph nodes. These dissections are generally submitted by the surgeon as separate specimens. Frequently, the decision to resect the prostate will depend on the presence or absence of metastatic carcinoma in these nodes. Consequently, you will need to become efficient at quickly identifying and examining these lymph nodes so that the presence or absence of significant metastasis can be established without undue delay.

Pelvic lymph node dissections consist of variable numbers of lymph nodes embedded in fibrofatty connective tissue. The identification of lymph nodes is greatly facilitated by the removal of perinodal fat. Without using excessive force, use your thumb to squeeze and liquefy the fat into absorbent paper towels. Once this excess fat has been removed, separate the lymph nodes so that each can be evaluated individually. Section the lymph nodes, and inspect their cut surfaces. Because normal pelvic lymph nodes are often scarred and fibrotic, it may be difficult to appreciate metastatic tumor nodules on visual inspection. Instead, metastases are firm and often can be detected by palpation. Each lymph node should be submitted for histologic evaluation. We also like to submit the remaining fat to search for microscopic soft tissue implants of metastatic carcinoma.

Important Issues to Address in Your Surgical Pathology Report on Radical Prostatectomies

- What procedure was performed, and what structures/organs are present?
- Where in the prostate is the bulk of the tumor located? Does it involve both sides of the gland?
- What are the histologic type and grade of the tumor?
- Does the tumor involve greater than 5% of the tissue resected?
- Does the tumor extend through the prostatic capsule? If so, where is the prostatic capsule penetrated by the tumor?
- Is vascular or perineural invasion identified?
- Does the tumor infiltrate the seminal vesicles?
- Is the tumor present at any of the following margins: proximal margin, distal margin, vasa deferentia margins, or soft tissue margins?
- Has the tumor metastasized to regional lymph nodes? Record the number of lymph node metastases and the total number of lymph nodes examined.

28 Testis

Biopsies

The most important thing to remember when processing a testicular biopsy is to treat it gently. The delicate sponge-like consistency of the testicular parenchyma makes it particularly susceptible to desiccation and compression. Be sure that the tissue remains in fixative during transportation and processing. Bouin's solution is a better fixative for these biopsies than is formalin. Take care not to crush the tissue when transferring the specimen to the tissue cassette. Do not use forceps; instead, gently filter the specimen into tissue paper. The entire specimen should be embedded and sectioned at multiple levels.

Radical Orchiectomies

When the entire testis is resected, it is usually removed in continuity with the epididymis and a variable length of the spermatic cord. Orchiectomy specimens can be oriented with relative ease using the epididymis as a landmark. The epididymis is roughly a C-shaped structure that cups the testis along its posterior aspect. Between the posterior aspect of the testis and epididymis is the mediastinum testis, where ducts, nerves, and vessels enter and exit the testis. The rete testis is a network formed in the mediastinum testis by the seminiferous tubules. Always be aware of the location of the mediastinum during your dissection because neoplasms and infections may extend beyond or into the testis at this site.

Weigh and measure the testis and epididy-mis, and also record the dimensions of the spermatic cord. The tunica vaginalis is a thin membranous sac that covers the external surface of the testis. After noting the appearance of its outer surface, open the tunica vaginalis along the anterior surface of the testis. Record the volume and appearance of any fluid that may have accumulated within this space, and examine the inner surface of the tunica for thickening or exophytic growths. The tunica albuginea is the thick fibrous capsule of the testis. Keep in mind that this resilient covering makes for an effective barrier to the diffusion of formalin and an equally formidable barrier to a dull knife. The testis should therefore be sectioned with a sharp knife before it is placed in fixative. As illustrated, partially bisect the testis along its long axis. Begin the cut along the anterior surface (the side opposite the epididymis), and extend the section into the mediastinum testis. The testis can now be opened much like a book with the epididymis serving as the bookbinding. This initial section will optimize your ability to assess the relationship between any focal lesions and the testicular parenchyma, the tunica vaginalis, and the epididymis. Furthermore, this section will allow formalin to penetrate and fix the testicular parenchyma. After making the initial section, photograph the specimen and collect tissue for special studies as indicated. A frozen section or touch preparation from the surface of the lesion may be used to determine if tissue needs to be sent for microbiologic studies, for a lymphoma workup, or for electron microscopy.

After the specimen is well fixed, it can be thinly sectioned at 3-mm intervals. Bread-loaf the testis along its long axis parallel to the initial section. The epididymis should be sectioned

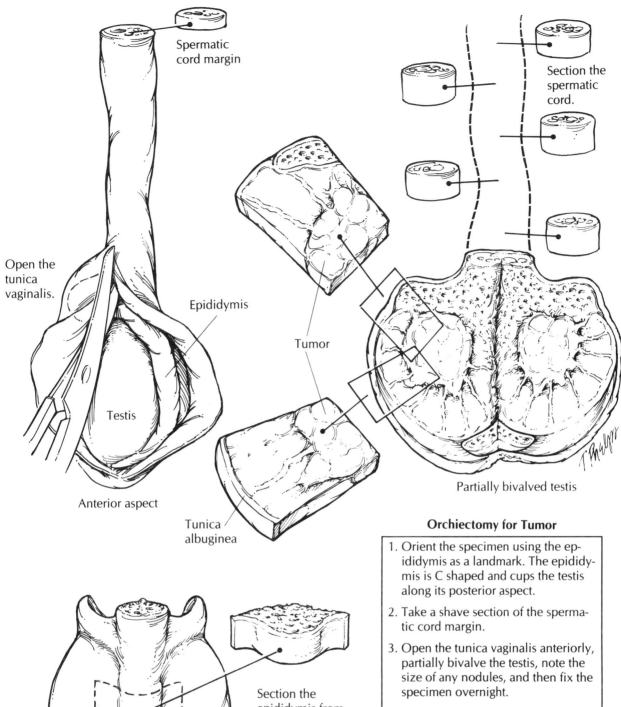

Spermatic cord margin

Section the spermatic cord.

Open the tunica vaginalis.

Epididymis

Tumor

Testis

Tunica albuginea

Anterior aspect

Partially bivalved testis

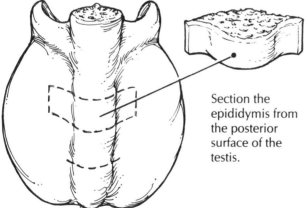

Section the epididymis from the posterior surface of the testis.

Posterior aspect

Orchiectomy for Tumor

1. Orient the specimen using the epididymis as a landmark. The epididymis is C shaped and cups the testis along its posterior aspect.

2. Take a shave section of the spermatic cord margin.

3. Open the tunica vaginalis anteriorly, partially bivalve the testis, note the size of any nodules, and then fix the specimen overnight.

4. Section the testis along its long axis parallel to the initial section. Section the epididymis from the posterior aspect of the specimen, perpendicular to its long axis.

5. Submit sections of tumor showing its relationship to the tunica albuginea, to the mediastinum testis, and to the testicular parenchyma. Submit sections of spermatic cord, of uninvolved testis, and of the epididymis.

151

from its head to its tail at right angles to its long axis. As illustrated, this is best accomplished from the posterior aspect of the specimen. Submit a shave section of the spermatic cord margin, and then serially section the remaining cord at regular intervals along its entire length.

Carefully examine the cut surface of the testis and paratesticular tissues. Give a detailed description of the appearance of any lesions, and try to determine their location (e.g., in the testis, epididymis, tunica vaginalis, or spermatic cord). When describing the appearance of a testicular mass, be sure to note its size and areas of hemorrhage and/or necrosis, even if these areas appear small and inconsequential. Try to determine if the tumor is confined to the testicular parenchyma, or if there is extratesticular extension, either beyond the tunica albuginea or into the epididymis. If a testicular neoplasm is clinically suspected, but one cannot be found on gross inspection, do not give up. Instead, scrupulously inspect the thin sections for any scars or areas of gritty calcification. These findings may represent regressive changes in a preexisting neoplasm.

The standard sections to be submitted from any orchiectomy specimen include: (1) sections of tumor showing its relationship to the tunica albuginea and to the mediastinum testis; (2) sections of the testicular parenchyma; (3) sections of the epididymis; (4) the spermatic cord margin; and (5) sections from three levels of the spermatic cord (i.e., proximal, mid, and distal). The number of sections that should be submitted is highly dependent on the clinical setting. Some of the more common reasons for which the testis is resected are cited below, along with some guidelines to keep in mind when sampling these specimens.

Sampling Testicular Neoplasms

Primary testicular neoplasms often exhibit more than one morphologic component (e.g., seminoma and embryonal carcinoma). Because even the focal presence of an aggressive component may impact on the treatment and prognosis, it is critical that all of the components present be demonstrated histologically. When submitting sections of primary testicular neoplasms, aim to be both thorough and selective. To be thorough, submit at least one section of tumor for every 1 cm of its greatest diameter. To be selective, sample the areas of the tumor that appear distinct on gross examination. For example, be sure to submit sections from areas of hemorrhage, necrosis, or mucinous change, even if these areas represent only a minor component of the tumor's gross appearance. These features often correlate with important histologic features.

Sometimes a primary testicular tumor can regress, leaving only a small scar. When a tumor cannot be identified in a testis removed from a patient with a metastatic germ cell tumor, the testis should be entirely submitted for microscopic examination.

Undescended Testis

The undescended testis is vulnerable to torsion, infarction, and most importantly, the development of germ cell neoplasms. Thus, a testis that is maldescended is often resected even when a tumor is not clinically apparent. Your principal role in the processing of the undescended testis is to determine if a neoplasm is present. Because early neoplastic changes or regressed tumors may not be apparent on gross examination, sample generously all areas of the testis even when a focal lesion is not seen. Just as in the normally positioned testis, an undescended testis removed from a patient with a metastatic germ cell tumor should be entirely submitted if a testicular tumor is not grossly apparent.

Bilateral Orchiectomies for Prostate Cancer

The testes removed from patients with metastatic prostatic carcinoma are not necessarily abnormal. Instead, bilateral orchiectomies in these patients are usually done as a therapeutic procedure to remove a source of testosterone. Nonetheless, carefully examine the specimen for a metastasis or an unsuspected primary tumor. If none is found, submit one section of the testicular parenchyma from each testis.

Torsion, Infarction, and Infectious Disease

For infectious processes, infarcts, and torsion, be sure to submit sections from both the periphery and the center of any lesions. The duration of testicular torsion and the host response to an infectious agent are best evaluated in the viable tissue at the periphery of a lesion. Also, when dealing with inflammatory lesions of the testis, always remember to submit fresh tissue for microbiologic studies.

Anorchia and Intersex Syndromes

Sometimes the pathologist is called on to determine the presence and/or type of gonadal tissue in a surgical specimen. In these instances, it is of critical importance that the specimen be reviewed and oriented with the surgeon. Label all of the grossly identifiable structures, and photograph the specimen so that the histologic findings can be correlated with the structures identified grossly. Always submit a section for histologic evaluation of each structure identified grossly. When the testis cannot be grossly identified, submit the entire tissue so that it can be evaluated for histologic evidence of testicular regression.

Important Issues to Address in Your Surgical Pathology Report on Orchiectomies

- What procedure was performed, and what structures/organs are present?
- Is a neoplasm present?
- Where does the tumor originate (i.e., testis, epididymis, spermatic cord)?
- What is the size of the tumor?
- What are the histologic type and grade of the neoplasm? Is intratubular germ cell neoplasia present?
- Is the tumor limited to the testis? Does the tumor extend into any of the adjacent structures: rete testis, epididymis, spermatic cord, tunica albuginea, or scrotum?
- Can vascular invasion be identified histologically?
- If a neoplasm cannot be identified, is there histologic evidence of intratubular germ cell neoplasia, calcification, or scar formation?
- Does the tumor involve any of the margins?

29 Kidney

General Comments

The gross examination plays an important role in the evaluation of kidney specimens. Macroscopic features often provide important clues to the underlying pathologic process. For example, the accurate pathologic staging of renal neoplasms can usually be accomplished simply by noting relationships between the tumor and certain anatomic landmarks. As with other tissues, no kidney specimen should be dissected without prior knowledge of the patient's clinical history. This fundamental rule is especially important when handling kidney specimens in which the evaluation of glomerular disease relies on immunofluorescence and ultrastructural analysis. Thus, before processing even the smallest kidney biopsy, determine from the clinical history whether or not fresh tissue should be submitted for these special studies.

Biopsies

Electron microscopy and immunofluorescence studies are central to the diagnostic evaluation of kidney biopsies for non-neoplastic disease. Even small specimens must be properly oriented because glomeruli should be included in the tissue submitted for each of these tests. The goal of orienting kidney biopsies is to distinguish cortex from medulla. While this distinction is usually quite simple with the larger wedge biopsies, the identification of cortex and medulla in small-needle biopsies often requires the use of a magnifying lens or dissection microscope. Under magnification, the cortex can be recognized by its red sunburst pattern corresponding to the vascular tufts of the glomeruli. In contrast, the straight vessels of the medulla are seen as thin red streaks coursing through tan/white tissue. From the tips of the cortical end, freeze a 1-mm section for immunofluorescence, and submit an adjacent 1-mm section in glutaraldehyde for electron microscopy. If multiple cores are received, do the same for each core. If you cannot confidently identify an end with cortex, do not guess. Rather, submit 1-mm sections from both ends of the core. For larger wedge biopsies, freeze a full-thickness section of cortex for immunofluorescence, and submit 1-mm cubes from the cortex in glutaraldehyde for electron microscopy. Submit the remainder of the tissue in fixative for routine histologic processing.

Nephrectomies for Neoplastic Disease

The purpose of evaluating kidneys resected for neoplasms is to determine the type of tumor, its extent, and the completeness of the resection. This can easily be achieved if you approach the nephrectomy as if it were made up of three individual compartments: the kidney, the renal hilum, and the perinephric fat. Describe each component of the kidney individually and systematically (Table 29-1).

First, weigh and measure the entire specimen. The renal capsule and the perinephric fat should not be stripped from the kidney until after their relationships to the tumor are established. Anatomically orient the specimen. The

Shave sections of the renal artery, renal vein, and ureteral margins.

Hilum

Bivalve the specimen.

Adrenal gland

Section of tumor, the renal capsule, and kidney

Section of tumor and perinephric fat

Gerota's fascia (the outer surface of the perinephric fat)

Normal kidney

Nephrectomy for Tumor

1. Use the ureter to orient the specimen. The ureter points to the inferior pole.

2. Shave the ureter, renal vein, and renal artery margins. Open and inspect the renal artery and vein.

3. Ink the perinephric fat soft tissue margins. Open the ureter, and bivalve the kidney.

4. Measure the size of the tumor, and try to assess if it is arising from the urothelium or renal parenchyma. Document any gross capsular invasion.

5. Submit sections to demonstrate the relationship of the tumor to the kidney parenchyma, renal pelvis, major blood vessels, renal capsule, and perinephric fat.

6. Submit sections of grossly normal kidney, sections of perinephric fat, a representative section of each lymph node, and sections of the adrenal gland.

155

ureter will provide a useful landmark: the downward course of the ureter points to the inferior pole of the kidney. By knowing whether the kidney is from the right or left side, you can then easily identify its anterior and posterior surfaces.

Begin the dissection at the kidney hilum. Identify the ureter, renal artery, and renal vein. Shave the margin from each, and then open each with a small pair of scissors to the point at which they enter the kidney. Look for the presence of vascular invasion, atherosclerosis, and thrombosis. Carefully inspect the mucosa and wall of the ureter. Is the ureter dilated or strictured? Are any masses present? Occasionally, lymph nodes will be present in the soft tissues of the hilum, and these should be individually measured and sampled. Other lymph node groups are usually submitted separately by the surgeon.

Next, ink the soft tissue margins and direct your attention to the dissection of the kidney itself. The objective of the initial section is to bivalve the kidney so that the relationship of the tumor to the kidney can be easily visualized. The plane of this initial section may vary depending on the location of the tumor, but in general it will be a sagittal cut that begins at the hilum and exits laterally through the perinephric fat. It may be helpful to insert probes into the calyces of the upper and lower poles of the kidney to guide the knife through the renal pelvis. Once the tumor is exposed, obtain fresh tissue for special studies such as electron microscopy, immunofluorescence, and cytogenetics, as is indicated. Photograph the bivalved specimen, and then submerge it in formalin until it is well fixed.

The outer surface of the fat represents Gerota's fascia. Ink this surface where it overlies the tumor, and submit perpendicular sections to show the relationship of the tumor to the soft tissue margin. Then carefully peel back the perinephric fat from the kidney, examine the capsular surface, and look for tumor extension through the renal capsule. Keep in mind that when renal tumors invade through the capsule, they tend to bulge from the surface of the kidney. Note any bulges, and document any disruption of the normal contour of the kidney surface by submitting sections that include the tumor, the adjacent non-neoplastic kidney, and the overlaying capsule. Make additional sections through the tumor, noting the appearance of its cut surface. Try to assess whether the tumor is arising from the urothelium or from the renal parenchyma.

Submit at least four sections of tumor (or more if necessary) to demonstrate the relationship of the tumor to the kidney parenchyma, renal pelvis, major blood vessels, renal capsule, and perinephric fat. Because some renal neoplasms are multifocal, section through the remainder of the kidney, looking for smaller tumors. Do not forget to describe the cortex, medulla, and collecting system of the nonneoplastic kidney. Also, submit one or two sections of the non-neoplastic kidney for histology.

TABLE 29-1. Non-neoplastic components of nephrectomy specimen to be inspected and described.

1. Hilum	
Vessels	• Patency (e.g., atherosclerotic plaque, thrombosis?)
Lymph nodes	• Number and size
Ureter	• Size (e.g., stenosis or dilatation?)
	• Appearance of mucosa (e.g., red, purulent?)
2. Kidney	
Capsular surface	• Contour (e.g., smooth, granular, coarsely scarred?)
	• Character of capsule (e.g., strips with ease, scarred, adherent?)
Cortex	• Thickness and color
Medulla	• Thickness and color
	• Shape of the pyramids
Collecting system	• Configuration (e.g., distortion, dilatation, stenosis)
	• Contents (e.g., stones)
	• Appearance of mucosa (e.g., red, purulent)
3. Perinephric fat	• Appearance
4. Adrenal gland	• Size and appearance

Finally, dissect the fibrofatty tissue enveloping the kidney, and submit one or two sections of the fat to assess infiltration by tumor.

Nephrectomy specimens often will include the adrenal gland. Be sure to look for it in the superior perinephric fat, and if it is present, weigh it, measure it, and submit a section. Keep in mind that the lymph nodes will be found in the soft tissues at the kidney hilum. A misdirected search for lymph nodes in the perinephric fat outside of the hilum will be a waste of your time.

Important Issues to Address in Your Surgical Pathology Report on Nephrectomies for Tumor

- What procedure was performed, and what structures/organs are present?
- Is a neoplasm present?
- Where is the tumor located?
- How large is the tumor?
- Does the tumor invade the renal capsule, Gerota's fascia, major veins, or the adrenal gland?
- What are the histologic type and grade of the neoplasm?
- What is the status of each of the margins (ureter, renal vein, soft tissue)?
- Are metastases identified? Record the number of nodes involved and the number examined.
- Does the non-neoplastic portion of the kidney show any pathology?

Partial Nephrectomies

Rarely, you may receive a partial nephrectomy—that is, a tumor removed with only a small portion of surrounding renal parenchyma. Take the same approach as you would for a total nephrectomy, only remember to sample the renal parenchymal margins. Ink these margins, and submit perpendicular sections to demonstrate the distance of the tumor's edge to the margin.

Nephrectomies for Non-neoplastic Disease

Dissection of the nephrectomy specimen is essentially the same for neoplastic and non-neoplastic diseases. Before beginning the dissection, try to establish from the patient's clinical history whether or not fresh cortical tissue should be taken for immunofluorescence studies or electron microscopy. Evaluate the kidney, the hilum, and the perinephric fat as three separate compartments, using the guidelines of dissection given earlier. When the specimen shows some modification (e.g., the absence of a perinephric soft tissue compartment), simply alter the dissection accordingly. Some pathologists may prefer to evaluate the texture of the cortical surface by stripping the capsule from the fresh specimen, and this can be done before the kidney is sectioned and fixed.

If calculi are identified during the dissection, submit some for chemical analysis if indicated. Because the macroscopic findings often provide crucial clues to the pathologic process involving the kidney, describe each component of the kidney individually and systematically (see table 29-1).

Cystic Kidneys

Sometimes kidneys are resected for congenital or acquired non-neoplastic cystic disease. Even for massively enlarged and distorted kidneys, the dissection should follow the same guidelines given above, only remember to pay particular attention to the following points: (1) Probe the ureters before opening them to check for patency; (2) Note the location of the cysts in terms of their relationship to the cortex and medulla; (3) Document the size and contents of the cysts; (4) Last, because cystic kidneys can harbor unsuspected neoplasms, thoroughly section and inspect the kidney. Submit sections of any suspicious areas, including solid foci, cysts with thickened walls, and cysts with a papillary surface.

30 Bladder

Biopsies

Biopsies of the urinary bladder are generally taken through the cystoscope. They vary from single and minute to numerous, large, and papillary. Orientation of these specimens is generally impossible, even for the larger papillary fragments. Biopsies of neoplasms potentially hold important information regarding tumor type, tumor grade, and extent of tumor invasion into the various layers of the bladder wall. By following two simple rules, you can avoid missing this crucial information. First, be sure to submit all of the pieces of tissue for processing and multiple sectioning. Second, avoid the common mistake of overfilling specimen cassettes with tissue fragments. Keep in mind that portions of the specimen will not be sampled if they are "buried" within a crowded cassette. In addition, we strongly recommend that the urologist submit superficial and deep tumor biopsies as separate specimens to facilitate the detection of deep muscle invasion.

Total Cystectomies

The processing of resected urinary bladders can be accomplished in three steps: (1) orientation of the specimen and identification of relevant structures (e.g., ureters); (2) fixation of the specimen; and (3) dissection of the specimen. Given the spherical shape of the bladder, this first step, orientation, is not necessarily an easy one. The peritoneum covering the surface of the bladder can be used as a reliable, though subtle, anatomic landmark. As illustrated, the perito-

neum descends further along the posterior wall of the bladder than it does along the anterior wall. If they are present, other pelvic organs can also be used to orient the specimen. For example, the seminal vesicles and uterus mark the posterior aspect of the bladder. Once the specimen is oriented, locate both ureters and, when present, the vasa deferentia. The best place to look for the ureters is in the lateral perivesicular fatty connective tissues. The ureters are much easier to locate and dissect in the fresh state than they are once the specimen is fixed. Tag the end of each ureter with a safety pin so that you can locate them later.

The next step is to fix the specimen. Some prefer to fix bladders in distention, either through the urethra via a catheter or through the bladder wall using a large-gauge needle. The method we prefer and describe below is to open the bladder and pin it out before submerging it in formalin. The advantage of this latter method is that by exposing the tumor before fixation, samples can be collected for ancillary studies requiring fresh tissue. Begin by inking the surface of the perivesicular soft tissues, and then open the anterior bladder wall from the urethra to the bladder dome using scissors. Avoid disrupting the posterior wall, because the ureteral orifices are located in this region, and they will serve as important anatomic landmarks later in the dissection. Examine the mucosa for ulcerations, exophytic tumors, or more subtle mucosal alterations. Note the size, gross morphology (flat, papillary, or ulcerated), and location (e.g., dome, trigone, free walls, etc.) of any lesions in the bladder. Photograph the opened specimen. Collect fresh tissue for special studies if warranted. Pin the specimen to a wax block such that the bladder cavity is opened and the luminal surface is fully exposed, and submerge the entire specimen in formalin.

After the specimen is well fixed, resume the dissection by shaving the margins from each of the ureters and (when present) the vasa deferentia. These already should have been located and tagged in the fresh specimen. The urethral margin should also be taken as a thin shave section. When the specimen includes the prostate (see below), this distal urethral margin should be taken from the distal end of the prostate. Next, using a small pair of scissors, open the ureters on both sides, beginning at their trigone orifices. Look for ureteral strictures and dilatations, and examine the mucosa for ulcerations or exophytic lesions. Document these findings in the gross dictation. Submit transverse sections of the ureters at regular intervals along their entire length.

If a tumor is identified in the bladder, try to determine its depth of invasion. To do this, make a full-thickness cut through the tumor and bladder wall. See whether or not the tumor appears to infiltrate the muscularis propria of the bladder and, if so, whether it extends into the surrounding soft tissues. Take sections of the tumor to demonstrate its relationship to the adjacent urothelium and, importantly, its maximal depth of invasion. Keep in mind that for large exophytic tumors sections will be more informative when they are taken from the base of the tumor than when they are taken from its surface.

Urothelial neoplasms often arise in a background of widespread epithelial alterations. Furthermore, many urothelial neoplasms are treated before surgical resection, and residual tumors may not be grossly apparent. For these reasons, it is important that bladders resected for urothelial neoplasia be extensively sampled for histology, even at sites that appear distant from the tumor. As a guide for sampling, treat the bladder as though it were a box with six walls including the floor (trigone), roof (dome), right and left lateral walls, anterior wall, and posterior wall. Submit two sections from each of these, as well as longitudinal sections through the ureteral orifices on both sides. Selectively sample areas where the mucosa appears abnormal. Carefully inspect the bladder mucosa because many *in situ* neoplasms of the bladder are flat and are characterized by a subtle red velvety appearance, which contrasts to the tan and smooth appearance of normal mucosa.

Section through the perivesicular soft tissues, and look for tumor extension beyond the bladder wall. Submit perpendicular sections from the soft tissue margins. Be sure to search for lymph nodes, which are sometimes present in the perivesicular soft tissues. If any are found, measure them individually, and submit a section of each for histologic evaluation.

Partial Cystectomies

Less frequently, only a portion of the bladder is removed as a sheet-like piece of tissue. In general, these partial cystectomies should be fixed and dissected according to the guidelines given for complete bladder specimens, keeping in mind that orientation of these specimens may not always be possible. Rather than a three-dimensional box, the partial cystectomy can be thought of as a rectangular sheet with four edges. These edges are important, because they represent the surgical margins of the bladder wall. Ink the edges and assess these margins for tumor involvement by taking perpendicular sections from all edges of the rectangle at regular intervals. Remember to include mucosa as well as the wall of the bladder in these sections.

A peculiar variation of the partial cystectomy is seen in resections of neoplasms arising from the urachal tract. These specimens consist of the dome of the bladder in continuity with the urachal tract up to and including the umbilicus. As illustrated, the bladder portion of the specimen should be routinely processed as you would any ordinary partial cystectomy. As for the urachal tract, first ink the surrounding soft tissue margins, and then serially section through the tract from the bladder to the umbilicus. These sections should be taken at right angles to the long axis of the urachal tract. Submit a number of these cross sections from the urachal tract for histology as well as the standard bladder sections. Remember to sample the two additional margins introduced by this resection: the soft tissue margin surrounding the urachus and the skin margin rimming the umbilicus.

En Bloc Resections

Commonly, the bladder is removed in continuity with the prostate, uterus, or other pelvic or-

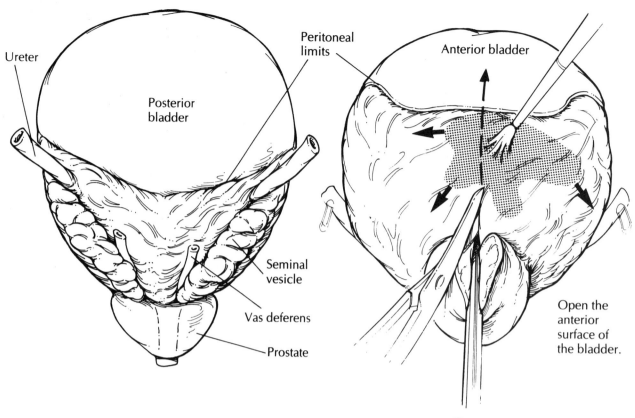

Ureter

Posterior
bladder

Peritoneal
limits

Seminal
vesicle

Vas deferens

Prostate

Anterior bladder

Open the
anterior
surface of
the bladder.

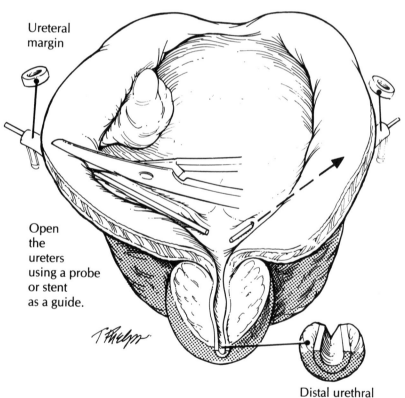

Ureteral
margin

Open
the
ureters
using a probe
or stent
as a guide.

T. Phelps

Distal urethral
margin

Cystoprostatectomy

1. Orient the bladder. The peritoneum extends further down the
   posterior wall than it does anteriorly.

2. Open the prostate and bladder
   along the anterior surface, beginning at the distal urethra.

3. Think of the bladder as a box with
   sides made up of the trigone,
   dome, anterior wall, posterior
   wall, left lateral wall, and the
   right lateral wall.

4. Submit shave sections of distal
   urethral and ureteral margins and
   perpendicular sections from the
   closest soft tissue margin.

5. Submit sections of the tumor to
   demonstrate its maximal depth of
   invasion and the relationship of
   the tumor to the bladder mucosa.
   Submit two sections of the trigone, dome, anterior wall, posterior wall, left lateral wall, and
   right lateral wall. Submit transverse sections of the ureters and a
   longitudinal section through the
   ureteral orifices. Include standard
   prostate sections. Submit sections
   of any lymph nodes.

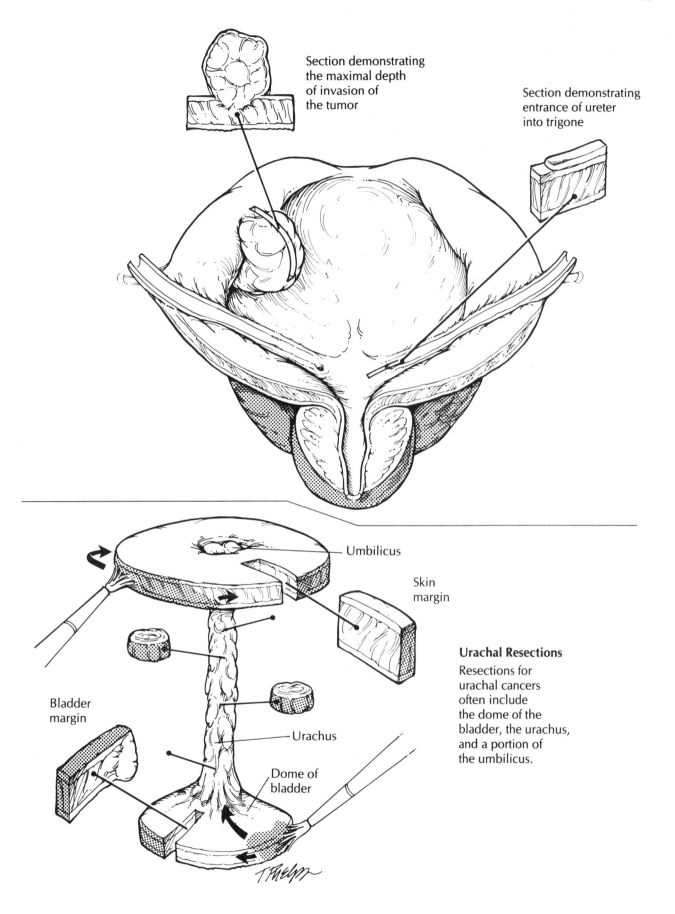

Section demonstrating the maximal depth of invasion of the tumor

Section demonstrating entrance of ureter into trigone

Umbilicus

Skin margin

Bladder margin

Urachus

Dome of bladder

Urachal Resections
Resections for urachal cancers often include the dome of the bladder, the urachus, and a portion of the umbilicus.

gans. The added complexity of these specimens introduces only minor alterations to the guidelines given above. For cystoprostatectomies, you will again need to open the specimen anteriorly before fixing it; only now begin the incision at the distal prostatic urethra. Using a pair of scissors, open the prostate anteriorly by cutting along the prostatic urethra, and continue the incision through the anterior bladder wall all the way to the dome. Try not to disrupt the posterior aspect of the prostate with this first longitudinal cut. After the specimen has been opened, carefully examine the urethral mucosa for evidence of extension of tumor into the prostatic urethra. Once the specimen is fixed, serially section the prostate from apex to base at 2- to 3-mm intervals. These sections should be transverse sections through the posterior surface of the gland. Examine the cut surface of the prostate. If a tumor is identified, try to determine if it is arising centrally from the prostatic urethra or if it is more peripherally located, as is common for cancer of the prostate. This observation is important, because the prostate should be processed differently (see Chapter 27) if a primary prostate carcinoma is present. If no peripheral tumors are noted, then a more limited sampling of the prostate is in order. These prostate sections should include: (1) shaved margins from the distal prostatic urethra and the vasa deferentia; (2) a posterior transverse section from the apical, mid, and basilar regions of the gland; (3) two cross sections of the prostatic urethra; and (4) a section of each seminal vesicle.

Because the other pelvic organs commonly removed with the bladder (e.g., uterus and rectum) are situated posteriorly, use the same anterior approach to open the bladder without altering its relationship to these other organs. Section these additional structures, keeping four objectives in mind: (1) document the presence of these structures; (2) demonstrate the relationship between the tumor and each of these structures; (3) evaluate the resection margins for each organ; and (4) examine the attached pelvic organs for other diseases. For example, when a portion of rectum accompanies the bladder specimen, sections should be submitted: (1) to document the presence of rectum and any incidental rectal pathologic findings; (2) to demonstrate the relationship between the rectum and the tumor; and (3) to assess the status of the proximal and distal rectal margins.

Important Issues to Address in Your Surgical Pathology Report on Cystectomies

- What procedure was performed, and what structures/organs are present?
- Is a neoplasm present?
- Where in the bladder is the tumor located (trigone, anterior wall, posterior wall, left lateral wall, right lateral wall, dome)?
- How large is the tumor?
- What is its pattern of growth? Is it papillary, flat, or ulcerated?
- Is the neoplasm *in situ* or infiltrating?
- What are the size, histologic type, and grade of the neoplasm?
- What is the maximal depth of invasion of the neoplasm? Does it extend into the lamina propria, the inner half of the muscularis propria, or the outer half of the muscularis propria?
- Does the tumor extend beyond the bladder into the perivesicular fat, prostate, uterus, vagina, pelvic wall, or abdominal wall?
- What is the status of each of the margins (the ureters, urethra, soft tissue, etc.)?
- Is the tumor multifocal or unifocal?
- Does the tumor involve blood vessels, nerves, or regional lymph nodes? How many lymph nodes were examined, and how many harbor a metastasis?

IX   The Ocular System

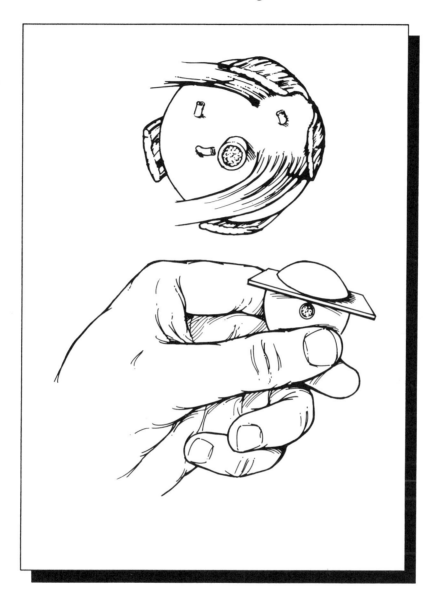

31 Eye

Robert H. Rosa, Jr., M.D., and W. Richard Green, M.D.

General Comments

The eye is a unique neurosensory organ. Much information can be gathered from the gross and microscopic examination of enucleated globes regarding the pathogenesis and manifestations of ocular and systemic diseases. In this chapter, we provide basic guidelines for the fixation and sectioning of ocular tissues, with emphasis on grossing the enucleated globe.

Enucleation Specimens

Fixation

The most commonly used fixative for ocular tissues is 10% neutral buffered formalin (4% formaldehyde), but even this standard fixative has its disadvantages. The relatively high osmolarity of 10% neutral buffered formalin may cause contraction of the anterior chamber and vitreous cavity, which may result in artifactual detachment of the retina. Moreover, formalin tends to dissolve water-soluble substances such as glycogen, resulting in shrinkage of fixed tissue. Thus, it is even a less suitable fixative when electron microscopy studies are required. The amount of 10% neutral buffered formalin required for adequate fixation varies with the size of the ocular specimen. For example, a small specimen such as a cornea or lid biopsy may require only 5 to 10 mL of formalin; an enucleated globe, 150 to 300 mL of formalin; and an orbital exenteration, 500 mL of formalin.

One alternative to formalin is glutaraldehyde 4%. This solution provides adequate fixation for both light and electron microscopy, while causing much less tissue shrinkage because of its lower osmolarity. For specimens less than 2 mm in diameter, glutaraldehyde 2% to 2.5% may be the preferred primary fixative for electron microscopy. Glutaraldehyde, however, causes tissues to become hard and brittle and may adversely affect the staining of tissues. For example, ocular tissues fixed in glutaraldehyde 4% stain less vividly with alcian blue and colloidal iron techniques, and they stain diffusely and nonspecifically with the periodic acid-Schiff (PAS) reaction. Yet another alternative is to combine fixatives to achieve optimal preservation for both light and electron microscopy. For example, a solution that combines 4% formaldehyde and 1% glutaraldehyde in 0.1 mol/L phosphate buffer can be used.

Fixation of ocular tissues requires patience. Practices that are designed to speed up the process (e.g., opening the globe, cutting windows into the sclera, or injecting fixative directly into the vitreous) are strongly discouraged because they are likely to induce artifactual disruption of the ocular tissues. The fixation of an enucleated globe in formalin generally requires 24 to 48 hours. After fixation, gently rinse the globe in running water for 16 hours, then place it in ethyl alcohol 60% for grossing.

Globes that contain excessive calcium deposits or even bone formation may require special decalcifying agents in addition to routine fixatives. In these cases, first fix the globe and then decalcify it in a solution of sodium citrate and formic acid for 24 to 72 hours. When the specimen is soft enough to section, wash it overnight in running tap water to remove all traces of acid, and then place the specimen in ethyl alcohol 60% before further processing. Because decalcification obscures histologic detail and interferes with staining, check the specimen daily while it is in solution to avoid excessive decalcification.

External Examination

Proper orientation of the globe is essential to document the location of a lesion within the eye. Although the globe is roughly spherical, careful attention to external landmarks allows one to orient this structure with respect to the horizontal median and nasal aspect. One such landmark is the cornea. The cornea occupies the anterior one sixth of the globe, measuring about 11 mm in its vertical plane and 11.5 mm in its horizontal plane. Thus, the longer axis of the cornea indicates the horizontal meridian. Other external landmarks are even more helpful in orienting the globe. The posterior ciliary arteries, for example, can be used to determine both the horizontal plane and the nasal aspect of the specimen. These vessels enter the sclera in the region of the optic nerve and then extend horizontally. Importantly, the nasal vessel is usually more prominent and therefore can be used to identify the nasal aspect of the globe. The nasal aspect can also be identified by measuring the distance between the limbus (the periphery of the cornea where it joins the sclera) and the optic nerve. This distance is shortest along the nasal aspect.

Perhaps the most reliable landmarks for orienting the eye are the insertions of the extraocular muscles. The use of these landmarks, however, requires a good understanding of ocular anatomy (Figure 31-1). The tendon of the superior oblique muscle extends temporally from the trochlea in the nasal orbital wall to insert into the sclera superotemporally posterior and just temporal to the superior rectus insertion and superior to the optic nerve. The inferior oblique muscle extends temporally from the inferonasal orbital wall to insert into the sclera (as a muscular rather than as a tendinous insertion) just temporal to the optic nerve and posterior ciliary vessel. The insertion of the inferior oblique muscle overlies an area of the sclera corresponding to the macula inside the eye.

Once the globe has been properly oriented, measure its anteroposterior, horizontal, and vertical dimensions. Record all measurements in millimeters. Also record the dimensions of the cornea and the length of the optic nerve stump. Describe any abnormal external features such as corneal opacities and lacerations or wounds of the cornea and/or sclera. A careful external examination will often disclose important information regarding a history of eye pathology. Scars located at the superior limbus may suggest prior surgery for cataracts or glaucoma, and the presence of a silicone band or sponge suggests prior surgery for retinal detachment. If these silicone bands and sponges are encountered, they need not be dislodged, because they will dissolve during processing. On the other hand, metal clips should be meticulously removed from any area submitted for histologic evaluation.

For cases of suspected melanoma, carefully examine the outer surface of the specimen for tumor spread. Specifically, examine the vortex veins for engorgement by tumor, check the episcleral soft tissues for pigment deposition, and look for gross extrabulbar extension by the tumor. In cases of suspected retinoblastoma, carefully examine the optic nerve grossly, and take the surgical margin of the optic nerve for microscopic examination. A dissecting microscope is extremely helpful in identifying minute lesions, and it should be employed during the external and intraocular examinations.

Photography plays an integral part of the gross examination of ocular tissues. As discussed in Chapter 3, photographs are useful for documenting any abnormal features of the external globe and are very helpful in correlating these gross features with the clinical findings. Likewise, photographs should be taken of intraocular lesions after the eye has been opened. The best photographs are obtained with the specimen submerged in alcohol (60%) and with even illumination.

Transillumination of the globe plays an important role in the localization of intraocular tumors that cannot be directly visualized on external examination. To transilluminate the specimen, place the eye in front of a small intense light against a dark background. One method is to use a substage microscope lamp in a dark room. Rotate the globe over the light source, and look for areas of increased or decreased transmission of light. Increased transmission of

Limbus

Pupil–optic nerve segment

Figure 31-1 (Top). The posterior external aspect of a normal right globe.

Figure 31-2 (Middle). Routine sectioning of the globe with horizontal cuts. The pupil, optic nerve, and macula are all in the same plane (see anterior and posterior views).

Figure 31-3 (Bottom). Sectioning of the globe with vertical cuts to incorporate the cataract scar into the pupil–optic nerve segment.

Cataract scar

Iridectomy

Tumor

Figure 31-4 (Top). Sectioning of the globe with oblique cuts to incorporate the area of a transillumination defect into the pupil–optic nerve segment.

Figure 31-5 (Middle). Alternate examination techniques for an eye with a melanoma anterior and posterior to the equator.

Figure 31-6 (Bottom). Sectioning of inferior or superior cap for histopathologic examination of a lesion in the peripheral retina.

Tumor posterior to equator

Tumor anterior to equator

Section the tumor transversely

Peripheral retinal lesion

Superior cap with a small V cut to help orient the tissue during embedding light may be seen in defects of the iris as occur in pigmentary dispersion syndrome and following peripheral iridectomy or cataract surgery. Decreased transmission of light may be due to intraocular hemorrhage or intraocular tumors. Mark these transillumination defects on the corresponding sclera with a pencil. The location of these transillumination defects will determine how the eye should be sectioned.

Sectioning

The planes of section through the globe depend on the presence and location of a lesion. Begin by cutting off the distal 3-mm portion of the optic nerve, and submit this portion on end for histologic examination. If no focal lesions are apparent after external examination, transillumination, and review of the clinical and surgical findings, open the eye in a horizontal plane parallel to the center of the optic nerve and macula. The ultimate aim is to provide a median section along the pupil and optic nerve axis—the pupil-optic nerve (P-O) section —which includes the pupil, optic nerve head, and macula in the same section. Approaching the globe from its posterior aspect, place a razor blade 5 mm superior to the center of the optic nerve. Do not aim the blade toward the center of the pupil, as the lens is a hard structure that is easily dislodged if you try to cut through it. Instead, avoid the lens by aiming 0.5 mm central to the limbus. Once the razor blade is engaged, turn the eye, and view it from the side to help maintain the proper plane of sectioning. Using a sawing motion, continue the section all the way through the limbus (Figure 31-2).

Before sectioning further, stop to examine the intraocular components. This examination should be performed with a dissecting microscope. Systematically evaluate the lens, iris, ciliary body, vitreous, choroid, retina, and optic nerve head. Note the size and location of any lesions. If an intraocular tumor is present, document its location using the ora serrata, optic disc, and macula as points of reference. Record its size in all dimensions. Try to determine which ocular structures are involved. Specifically note the relationship of the tumor to the optic nerve.

Once the intraocular examination is complete, finish sectioning the eye. Place the cut surface of the globe on a flat surface, and then cut the eye in a plane parallel to the initial section. Again, the razor blade should enter the posterior aspect of the eye 5 mm from the center of the optic nerve, and it should exit the anterior surface of the eye through the periphery of the cornea (i.e., 0.5 mm central to the limbus). The completion of this second cut will result in two caps (or callottes) and the P-O segment.

For globes with focal lesions, the globe can be sectioned vertically or obliquely to include the lesion in the P-O plane. A few common examples are worthy of specific description. If evidence of prior cataract surgery is present, cut the globe vertically in a plane perpendicular to the wound (Figure 31-3). If a corneal laceration is present, cut the globe perpendicular to the long axis of the lesion. If a transillumination defect (e.g., melanoma) is present, cut the globe so that the center of the tumor is in the plane of the P-O segment (Figure 31-4).

An alternative technique for sectioning an eye with melanoma has been designed to permit direct visualization of the tumor from the perspective of the clinician and thus enhance clinicopathologic correlations.[5] For melanomas located posterior to the equator, the anterior segment (cornea, iris, lens, and pars plicata) is removed en bloc by a coronal cut through the pars plana just anterior to the ora serrata. For melanomas that extend anterior to the equator, a cap is removed by a cut along the P-O plane. Either of these cuts permits the examiner to look into the globe and directly visualize the apex of the tumor (Figure 31-5).

Tissue Sampling

In most cases, only the P-O segment is submitted for histologic evaluation. Important exceptions are when a cap contains the macula (as when the P-O segment is taken in the vertical plane) or a lesion. If a lesion is present in the cap, then the cap may be further sectioned into superonasal, superotemporal, inferonasal, and/or inferotemporal segments, as necessary, and submitted for processing. A mark on the tissue section and a note to the histotechnologist may help guide proper orientation of the tissue during embedding. For example, a small V may be cut into the segment opposite the margin of interest with instructions provided to ''embed V up'' (Figure 31-6). The pathologist may wish to supervise the embedding of the tissue to ensure proper orientation. Store any remaining tissue in formalin, taking care to designate the tissue properly.

Cataract Specimens

The handling of cataract specimens varies from institution to institution. In general, cataracts are difficult to evaluate by light microscopy. Hence, the histopathologic examination of cataract specimens is performed only for special indications (such as with congenital cataracts and pseudoexfoliation syndrome). If the submission of cataract specimens is required, document the color, diameter, and thickness of the lens nucleus.

Intracapsular cataract extraction (ICCE) is a surgical technique that allows for the best evaluation of the lens, as the lens is removed in its entirety (capsule, cortex, and nucleus). ICCE was the procedure of choice for cataract extraction for many years; however, this technique is used today only in rare circumstances (such as in conditions with zonular weakness).

Phacoemulsification is a type of small-incision extracapsular cataract extraction (ECCE) that was initially introduced in 1967. Recently, this technique has gained popularity over the more traditional technique of ECCE. With phacoemulsification, there is a smaller incision, less induced astigmatism, and perhaps a faster recovery of vision. The lens nucleus is emulsified ultrasonically; therefore, no cataract specimen is submitted.

Eyelid Excisions

Basal cell carcinoma accounts for 85% to 95% of all malignant epithelial tumors of the eyelids. Most excised specimens with basal cell carcinoma are elliptical. If the long axis of the specimen is less than 10 mm, the specimen should be bisected perpendicular to its long axis through the center of the tumor. This technique allows for the evaluation of three surgical margins (two skin margins and the deep margin). If the ellipse is larger than 10 mm, the specimen can be cut in a cruciate configuration, resulting in a 3- to 4-mm central portion and two end portions.

The two end portions are bisected in a plane perpendicular to the central portion. Separately label and submit the central portion and end sections. With this technique, all five surgical margins (e.g., deep, lateral, medial, superior, and inferior) are evaluated.

Special Techniques

Given the easy accessibility of the eye, small tissue samples for diagnostic purposes are readily obtained using a variety of methods. Although these specimens do not require complex dissections, they do require careful handling to preserve cellular detail. Scrapings of the cornea and conjunctiva can be processed as wet-fixed smears. This technique is useful in cases of conjunctival intraepithelial neoplasia. Rapid fixation of the slides in 95% ethyl alcohol is essential in this technique. Do not allow the specimen to air dry. After fixation, the slides may be stained with a modified Papanicolaou technique. Air-dried smears are often useful to look for infectious agents in cases of suspected exogenous or endogenous endophthalmitis. Drops of the specimen are placed on the center of three or more slides and allowed to air dry. The slides can then be fixed in 100% methanol for 5 minutes. Microorganisms can then be detected using Gram, Giemsa, PAS, and Papanicolaou stains.

The Millipore filter preparation technique can be used to examine ocular fluid specimens in cases of vitreous hemorrhage, proliferative vitreoretinopathy, and suspected intraocular tumors. This procedure provides for excellent cytologic preservation. The specimen may be received in a plastic syringe or a vitrectomy cassette and must be fresh and unfixed before filtration. After filtration, the cells are fixed with 95% ethyl alcohol. Do not allow the filter to air dry at any time during the procedure. If a specimen is very cellular, divide it among several filters. During filtration, direct the washings along the sides of the funnel to avoid disturbing the cells on the filter. Fix the filters for a minimum of 15 minutes in a Petri dish with 95% ethyl alcohol. A modified Papanicolaou technique, Gomori's stain for iron, and the PAS stain are routinely used to stain the Millipore filter. Absolute propyl alcohol rather than absolute ethyl alcohol should be used during staining to avoid dissolution of the filter. The stained Millipore filters are then mounted on glass slides for microscopic examination.

The celloidin bag technique is useful for the retrieval of tissue fragments and cellular material suspended in a fluid. Place 10% neutral buffered formalin and the specimen into a centrifuge tube lined by a celloidin bag. Centrifuge for 10 minutes. Decant the supernatant, remove the celloidin bag, and tie the bag with a string just above the pellet. Fix the specimen again in formalin for at least 30 minutes. The specimen may now be submitted for routine paraffin processing and sectioning.

Important issues to Address in Your Surgical Pathology Report on the Eye

- What procedure was performed?
- Is the specimen a right or left eye? What is the size of the globe? (What are the anteroposterior, horizontal, and vertical dimensions? What is the length of the optic nerve? What are the horizontal and vertical dimensions of the cornea?)
- What is the status of the anterior segment (surgical incisions, corneal opacification, iris or lens abnormalities)?
- Are any transillumination defects present? What are the measurements of these defects, and where are they in relation to external landmarks?
- Note the condition of the iris, ciliary body, and lens. Is an intraocular lens present? If so, is it in the anterior or posterior chamber? If in the posterior chamber, is it in the capsular bag or in the sulcus (between the ciliary body and the root of the iris)?
- Is there a posterior vitreous or retinal detachment? Is any hemorrhage present in the vitreous or retina? Is the choroid thickened? Is the optic nerve head cupped or swollen?
- Is an intraocular tumor present? Describe its type, location, size, color, margins, and consistency. Is any associated hemorrhage or necrosis present? What ocular structures are involved? Does the tumor extend into the optic nerve? Is the tumor present grossly at the cranial or surgical margin of the optic nerve?

X The Endocrine System

32 Thyroid

Thyroidectomies

One major task of the surgical pathologist evaluating a thyroid specimen is to identify the infrequent thyroid neoplasm from among the vast majority of harmless thyroid nodules—an effort that is shared with the cytopathologist, endocrinologist, and surgeon. Thorough inspection and appropriate sampling of the thyroid is central to the diagnosis and subsequent treatment of thyroid lesions.

The thyroid gland has a relatively simple anatomy. As illustrated, its shape resembles that of a butterfly with open wings: two expanded lateral lobes are bridged at the midline by the isthmus. In some specimens, a small triangular-shaped midline lobe (i.e., the pyramidal lobe) is also present. When present, the pyramidal lobe extends superiorly from the isthmus. The two most common resections of the thyroid are the total thyroidectomy, in which the entire gland is removed intact, and the hemithyroidectomy, in which a single lobe is removed by an incision through the isthmus. Orientation of these specimens is seldom problematic. The isthmus can be used to identify the inferior and medial aspects of the gland, and the posterior surfaces of the lateral lobes have a concave shape caused by the trachea.

Once the specimen has been oriented, it should be weighed and measured. Describe its shape, contours, and symmetry. Be sure to note the presence and appearance of any extrathyroidal tissues. In particular, inspect the posterior aspect of the specimen for parathyroid glands and lymph nodes, and inspect the anterior aspect for fragments of adherent skeletal muscle. Palpate the specimen to assess the consistency of the thyroid and to localize any focal lesions before cutting the specimen.

Paint the outer surfaces of the thyroid with ink, and in the case of the hemithyroidectomy, remove the isthmic margin as a thin shave section. Although the specimen can be serially sectioned in either the coronal, sagittal, or transverse plane, the relationship of a focal lesion to the thyroid capsule is often best demonstrated by cutting perpendicular to the long axis of each individual lobe. Once the thyroid is sectioned, sequentially lay out the individual slices in such a way as to maintain the proper orientation of the specimen.

Carefully inspect the cut surfaces of the specimen. Assess whether the thyroid is diffusely or focally abnormal. For diffuse lesions, ask yourself the following questions: Is the gland symmetrically or asymmetrically involved? Is the lesion confined to the thyroid, or does it extend beyond the capsule of the thyroid into the surrounding soft tissues? Is the lesion cystic, soft, firm, or hard? If an isolated lesion is identified, record its size and location, and determine if it is surrounded by a capsule. Keep in mind that the presence of a discrete nodule does not exclude the presence of additional lesions. Always look for multifocal lesions. Gentle palpation of each slice will sometimes reveal small but firm carcinomas that are not apparent simply by looking at the cut surface.

Imprints of the tumor allow quick and easy evaluation of its cytologic features and will nicely supplement the histologic findings of a

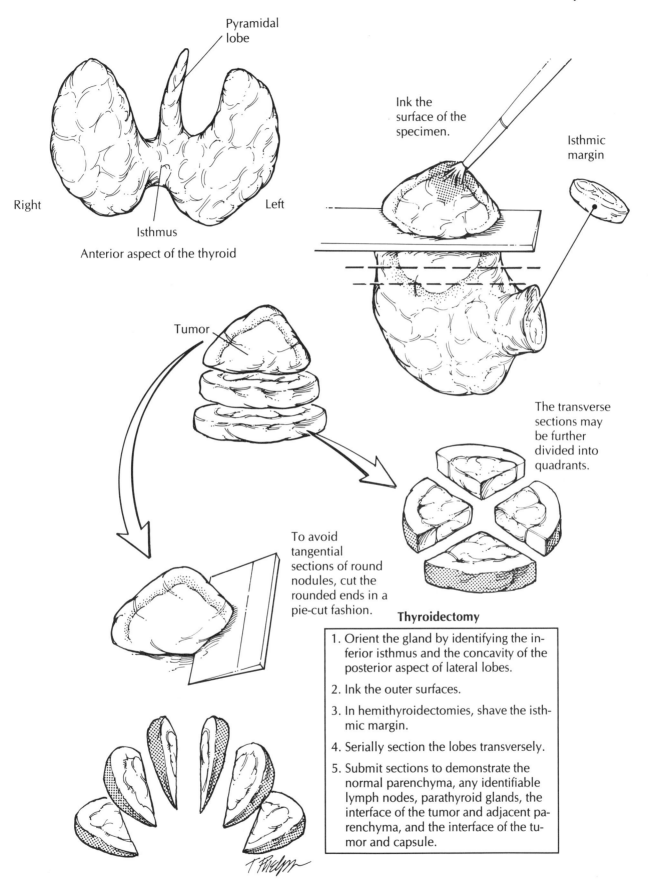

Pyramidal lobe

Isthmus

Right

Left

Anterior aspect of the thyroid

Ink the surface of the specimen.

Isthmic margin

Tumor

The transverse sections may be further divided into quadrants.

To avoid tangential sections of round nodules, cut the rounded ends in a pie-cut fashion.

Thyroidectomy

1. Orient the gland by identifying the inferior isthmus and the concavity of the posterior aspect of lateral lobes.

2. Ink the outer surfaces.

3. In hemithyroidectomies, shave the isthmic margin.

4. Serially section the lobes transversely.

5. Submit sections to demonstrate the normal parenchyma, any identifiable lymph nodes, parathyroid glands, the interface of the tumor and adjacent parenchyma, and the interface of the tumor and capsule.

frozen section. Simply touch the surface of a glass slide to the cut surface of the tumor, or smear a small piece of the tumor between two slides, and immediately fix the slides in 95% alcohol. These slides can be used for Diff-Quik or hematoxylin and eosin staining.

Sections for histology should be taken to demonstrate the following: (1) all components of a lesion (e.g., solid areas and cystic areas); (2) the interface of the tumor (and its surrounding capsule) with the adjacent non-neoplastic thyroid parenchyma; (3) the relationship of the tumor to the thyroid capsule and extrathyroidal soft tissues; and (4) the presence of parathyroids, lymph nodes, and normal-appearing thyroid parenchyma (one to two sections from each lobe). Since the histologic evaluation will be hampered if the tissue blocks are thick and bulky, fix the slices in formalin until they are firm enough to section thinly. Although these general guidelines should direct the sampling of any thyroid lesions, two frequently asked questions deserve special consideration:

1. *How many sections do I need to submit to avoid sampling error?* This question often arises in cases of multinodular goiters and encapsulated nodules. In multinodular goiters, the thyroid is often massively enlarged, and its cut surface may show numerous nodules, hemorrhage, calcification, scarring, and even necrosis. In these instances, try to avoid the common error of submitting too many sections. Instead, document the finding with a photograph and a detailed gross description. Sampling a multinodular goiter should be limited to one or two sections selectively taken from the periphery of each nodule (up to five nodules). Conversely, the more common error when sampling encapsulated nodules is to submit too few sections. Your primary task in sampling these lesions is to make sure that areas of transcapsular or vascular invasion are not missed. Since these areas usually cannot be seen by the naked eye, they can easily be missed unless the peripheral portion of the nodule is extensively sampled. The more capsule sampled, the greater chance of finding invasive foci. Therefore, the tumor–capsule–thyroid interface of any encapsulated nodule should be submitted in its entirety for histologic evaluation.

Similarly, thyroids removed from patients with one of the multiple endocrine neoplasia (MEN) syndromes should be extensively sampled for histology.

2. *How can I avoid tangential sections of a round nodule?* Tangential sections through a round nodule may give the artifactual microscopic impression that the tumor infiltrates the capsule. Whereas tangential sectioning is usually not a problem at the equator of a nodule where the knife easily passes perpendicular to the tumor capsule, it becomes increasingly difficult to avoid as one approaches the rounded ends of the nodule while bread-loafing the specimen. One method to minimize tangential sectioning is to cut these rounded ends like a pie rather than a loaf of bread.[6] Decapitate the rounded ends from the tumor nodule, place the flat surface of each end on the cutting board, and then, as illustrated, direct each cut perpendicular to the tumor capsule as though you were dividing a pie into equal pieces.

Regional neck lymph nodes are usually removed separately by the surgeon and submitted as separate specimens. These should be anatomically oriented, and each level should be carefully dissected (see Chapter 7 on radical neck dissections). A representative section of each lymph node identified should be submitted for histologic evaluation.

Important Issues to Address in Your Surgical Pathology Report on Thyroidectomies

- What procedure was performed, and what structures/organs are present?
- What is the size of the lesion, and where is it located?
- What are the histologic type and grade of the tumor (e.g., follicular, papillary, anaplastic, etc.)?
- For encapsulated neoplasms, does the tumor infiltrate blood vessels and/or its surrounding capsule?
- Is the lesion confined to the thyroid, or does it extend beyond the thyroid capsule into the extrathyroidal soft tissues?
- Are any abnormalities present in the non-

neoplastic thyroid tissue (e.g., goiter, lymph-ocytic thyroiditis, C-cell hyperplasia, etc.)?
- Is evidence of metastatic disease present? Record the number of lymph nodes with metastases and the total number of lymph nodes examined.

33 Parathyroid Glands

Parathyroidectomies

Parathyroid glands are usually removed from patients with hypercalcemia. During the removal of these glands, the surgeon often needs help identifying parathyroid tissue, determining whether the parathyroid tissue is proliferative, and distinguishing between hyperplasia involving multiple glands and a neoplasm confined to a single gland. For the surgical pathologist, these issues translate into two simple questions that can be promptly addressed: (1) Is parathyroid tissue present? (2) How large is the parathyroid gland?

1. *Is it parathyroid tissue?* Parathyroid glands are oval-shaped and encapsulated nodules that have a homogenous red-brown cut surface. This gross appearance of the parathyroid is not specific and may resemble a lymph node or a thyroid nodule. Fortunately, this distinction can be made with speed and relative ease by resorting to frozen section evaluation and/ or with a touch imprint from the surface of the encapsulated nodule.
2. *How big is it?* Perhaps the biggest oversight when evaluating parathyroid tissue is forgetting to weigh the tissue. While histologic examination is important in confirming the presence of a parathyroid gland, the histologic findings may not reliably distinguish between normal and proliferative parathyroid tissue. Instead, this distinction is best made by weighing the gland. Therefore, it is critical that every specimen potentially representing parathyroid tissue be accurately weighed. Once an enlarged parathyroid gland is removed, remain alert. Remember to weigh additional specimens, since their size may be critical in distinguishing between an isolated adenoma and diffuse hyperplasia.

With these two questions in mind, the dissection of parathyroid tissue is simple. Parathyroids are usually received from the operating room with a request for a frozen section evaluation to confirm the presence of parathyroid tissue. Measure and weigh the specimen, and note its gross appearance including its shape and color. Use a scale that is accurate to the nearest milligram. Sometimes, instead of a grossly apparent parathyroid gland, you may receive a portion of thyroid or thymus. Because the parathyroid may lie hidden deep in the parenchyma of these organs, they should be rapidly yet thoroughly dissected and inspected. In these cases, weigh the entire specimen before dissecting it, and then weigh the potential parathyroid gland alone once any associated tissues have been delicately removed. Bisect the parathyroid, and note the appearance of its cut surface. Touch imprints of the cut surface of the specimen (immediately fixed in 95% alcohol and stained with hematoxylin and eosin) can be used to differentiate parathyroid from thyroid and lymphoid tissue, and they often serve as a valuable adjunct to the frozen section.

In addition to the parathyroid gland, remember to sample other tissues that may be part of the specimen (e.g., thyroid gland, thymus, and associated soft tissues). Indeed, when these structures are removed in a search for an occult parathyroid gland, the entire specimen should be submitted for histologic evaluation if the parathyroid gland is not grossly apparent. In the rare case of a parathyroid carcinoma, sections should be submitted in an attempt to document local invasion by the tumor. These sections should demonstrate the relationship of the tumor to its capsule and to any adjacent structures (e.g., thyroid gland).

Important Issues to Address in Your Surgical Pathology Report on the Parathyroid

- What procedure was performed, and what structures/organs are present?

- Is parathyroid tissue present?
- What is the weight of the parathyroid gland (to the nearest milligram)?
- Based on the comparative weights and histologic features, is the tissue most consistent with normal parathyroid tissue, multiglandular hyperplasia, or an adenoma?
- For parathyroid carcinomas: What is the size of the carcinoma? Does the carcinoma extend beyond the tumor capsule? Is angiolymphatic invasion present? Does the carcinoma infiltrate into adjacent soft tissues and/or the thyroid? Are the margins involved by tumor?

34 Adrenal Glands

Adrenalectomies

Extrinsic hormonal influences and intrinsic pathologic processes have profound and predictable effects on the size, color, and shape of the adrenal gland. For example, the pathogenesis of hypercortisolism is frequently suggested by the size and color of the adrenal cortex, and the distinction between benign and potentially malignant cortical neoplasms is often based on the dimensions and weight of the tumor. Therefore, careful examination of the gross specimen plays an important role in recognizing and interpreting pathologic processes involving the adrenal gland.

A thorough evaluation of the specimen requires a certain familiarity with the anatomy and weight of the normal adrenal gland. As illustrated, the right adrenal gland has the shape of a pyramid, and the left adrenal gland, the shape of a crescent. The average weight of each is approximately 4 g in the adult. Weights of 6 g or more are abnormal. Specimen orientation is easily achieved by locating the concave surface of the specimen. This concavity is the point at which the adrenal abuts the ipsilateral kidney, and thus it represents the inferolateral aspect of the specimen. The adrenal gland is considered a tripartite structure composed of a head, body, and tail. The head is the thickest and broadest portion of the adrenal, and is situated most medially. The middle third represents the body. The thinnest and most lateral third represents the tail. Unlike the kidney, blood does not enter the adrenal at a single vascular pedicle. Instead, numerous small arteries pierce the cortex at multiple sites. Most of these vessels are too small to appreciate grossly. In contrast, the adrenal is drained by a single vein. This vein exits the adrenal at the junction of the body and the head of the gland and is usually visible to the naked eye, especially when filled and distended by tumor.

Examine the contours of the adrenal gland. Be sure to ink the soft tissues overlying any areas where tumor bulges from the surface of the adrenal, since these areas represent soft tissue margins. Look for and sample the adrenal vein. The entire specimen should then be measured and weighed. If the gland appears enlarged, determine and document whether this enlargement is due to a solitary mass, multiple nodules, or diffuse hyperplasia. Extended resections of primary adrenal tumors may also include portions of adjacent kidney, liver, and/or abdominal wall. The presence and appearance of these structures should be noted, and their relationships to the adrenal tumor should be described.

Serially section the adrenal gland at 3-mm intervals perpendicular to the long axis of the specimen. Keep in mind that although the adrenal gland is removed as a single structure, it is both structurally and functionally compartmentalized into a steroid-secreting cortex and a chromaffin-positive medulla. This compartmentalization will become most apparent when the adrenal is sectioned. The medulla is seen as an inner gray or white band confined mostly to the head of the adrenal. This central band is sharply demarcated from the outer yellow-brown cortex. The inner zone of the cortex is typically brown, while the outer zone of the cortex is often yellow. The inner zone corresponds to the lipofuscin-laden zona reticularis and the outer zone to the lipid-laden zona glomerulosa

Relative sizes of the cortex and medulla

Medulla   Cortex

Head

Adrenal vein

Body

Tail

Tumor

Section the adrenal in a plane perpendicular to the long axis.

Inferior vena cava

Aorta

Left kidney

Right kidney

Adrenalectomy

1. Orient the specimen. The concave surface of the adrenal represents the infero-lateral aspect of the gland.

2. Weigh the specimen, and document the size of any nodules.

3. Ink the specimen, and section it perpendicular to the long axis of the gland.

4. Measure the thickness of the cortex and medulla in the head, body, and tail.

5. Submit sections of the tumor to show its relationship to the capsule and to the adjacent adrenal tissue.

6. Submit sections of grossly uninvolved adrenal tissue.

and zona fasciculata. Measure and record the thickness of these compartments at three levels—the head, body, and tail. Remember to document the exact dimensions of any tumors and to record the appearance of the tumor's cut surface: What is its color? Is it necrotic and/or hemorrhagic? Is it encapsulated? Does it extend beyond the adrenal and into adjacent tissues?

Before the specimen is fixed in formalin, ask yourself if fresh tissue should be specially processed. For example, adrenal cortical neoplasms are sometimes evaluated for steroid content. Viable fresh tissue from these tumors can be snap frozen in liquid nitrogen and stored in a −70°C freezer for easy retrieval if tissue is later needed for biochemical analysis. Fresh tissues from adrenal medullary neoplasms have historically been processed in dichromate fixatives (e.g., Zenker's solution) to preserve cytoplasmic chromaffin granules. Today, this practice has limited value because these same catecholamines can be more precisely characterized and quantified from the patient's serum. Perhaps the strongest indication for special tissue processing is if the tumor was resected from a young patient. For adrenal tumors from pediatric patients—where a primitive neuroblastic tumor is often suspected—fresh tissue should be set aside for cytogenetic, molecular (e.g., N-myc amplification), and ultrastructural analysis (see Chapter 35 on pediatric neoplasms).

Sections from a tumor should be taken to demonstrate the relationship of the tumor to the adrenal, to the tumor capsule, and to any associated soft tissues and visceral organs. Do not forget to take sections from the surgical margins, including an appropriate margin from all structures represented in the extended resection (e.g., abdominal wall, kidney, etc.) and from the periadrenal fat overlying a bulging tumor. Large adrenal tumors should be sampled to include all components contributing to its often variegated appearance on cut section. For the uninvolved adrenal gland and for specimens that do not have a discrete lesion, submit a representative section from the head, body, and tail. To best demonstrate the cortex and medulla, these sections should be taken perpendicular to the long axis of the gland.

Regional lymph nodes will generally not be found in the specimen but will be separately submitted by the surgeon. Any lymph nodes that are present should, of course, be sampled for histologic evaluation.

Important Issues to Address in Your Surgical Pathology Report on Adrenalectomies

- What procedure was performed, and what structures/organs are present?
- What are the dimensions and weight of the adrenal gland?
- For focal tumors: From which compartment (cortex or medulla) does the tumor appear to arise? What are the dimensions and weight of the tumor? Does the tumor infiltrate vessels, the tumor capsule, and/or the surrounding tissues? What is the status of the surgical margins? Has the tumor metastasized to regional lymph nodes?
- For diffuse processes: Which compartment (cortex or medulla) is expanded? Is the compartment uniformly enlarged, or is the enlargement due to multiple nodules?

XI   Pediatric Tumors

35 Pediatric Tumors

Elizabeth J. Perlman, M.D.

General Comments

A number of tumors are unique to children. These tumors frequently require special processing to ensure that the diagnosis can be established and appropriate treatment given. Two large organizations in the United States create, monitor, and evaluate therapeutic protocols for pediatric tumors. These are the Pediatric Oncology Group and the Children's Cancer Study Group. Most hospitals that treat childhood tumors are affiliated with one of these groups. These groups frequently require that pathologic material be sent to review pathologists, to verify the diagnosis, and to further classify the tumor. These groups also often require that additional fresh and frozen tissue be harvested for biologic studies, which are performed at specialized reference laboratories. If this tissue is not collected at the time of surgery, the patient may not be eligible for the appropriate treatment protocol. Furthermore, as knowledge is accumulated and protocols change, tissue requirements may change. Therefore, pathologists who are processing pediatric tumors need to work closely with their pediatric oncologists to be aware of the current protocol requirements. Conversely, the entire specimen cannot be submitted for biologic studies. Sufficient tissue must be available to establish a histologic diagnosis. It is vital that the pathologist be responsible for the appropriate triage of this tissue, particularly because in many cases, tissue also needs to be submitted for ancillary diagnostic studies (such as electron microscopy and cytogenetics). Despite these demands, pediatric tumors can be processed easily if a series of steps is routinely performed at the time of initial processing. This is particularly important to remember because many biopsies are taken during off-hours.

Overall Guidelines

1. Ensure that *all* pediatric tumors are promptly received in the fresh state. This may entail processing during off-hours by on-call personnel.
2. Decide how much of the specimen is needed for routine histology. This will depend on the tumor type suspected and the size of the biopsy.
3. Submit tissue for electron microscopy. It is a good practice to put a small piece of every pediatric tumor in glutaraldehyde. This can then be embedded, and the decision of whether or not to section and process can be made at a later time.
4. Place ½ to 1 cc of minced tumor in Roswell Park Memorial Institute medium (RPMI) or equivalent tissue culture medium and refrigerate. This material can be submitted for cytogenetic analysis (if submitted to the laboratory within 24 hours) or mailed to a reference laboratory for special studies (such as ploidy, gene amplification studies, or fluorescence in situ hybridization).
5. Freeze 1 cc of tumor tissue in liquid nitrogen. This can be submitted to reference laboratories for protocol studies or held locally in a tumor bank if available. Normal tissue should also be frozen. If you have limited tissue, remember that the frozen section control is often inadequate for permanent histology, yet if it is kept frozen, it can be used for these studies.

Small Blue Cell Tumors of Childhood

Pediatric tumors are often embryonal neoplasms showing little or no differentiation by routine histology. In particular, at time of frozen section, these tumors appear to be primitive, small, round blue cell tumors. Their diagnosis often depends on ancillary studies such as immunohistochemistry, electron microscopy, and cytogenetics. If all pediatric specimens are processed as delineated in the first section, all necessary information should be available in a timely fashion. Table 35-1 lists the most common small blue tumors of childhood and their pertinent diagnostic parameters.

Pediatric Renal Neoplasms[7]

Pediatric renal tumors are often primarily resected and must be carefully processed to ensure accurate staging. Since these tumors are often bulky and friable and are therefore easily distorted, processing must be undertaken with care. (Refer also to Chapter 29, "Kidney".)

1. Photograph the nephrectomy specimen before bivalving. Carefully examine the contour of the kidney and the tumor, and identify potential sites of capsular penetration.
2. Ink the surface (do not strip the capsule).
3. Bivalve the specimen. The kidney should always be bivalved by the pathologist *after* steps 1 and 2 are performed, not by the surgeon and not in the operating room. Choose your plane of incision carefully, as the placement of the original incision determines your ability to document the relationship between the tumor and kidney, the tumor and the renal sinus, etc. The incision should be at or near the vertical midplane of the kidney. This cut should avoid sites of capsular penetration if possible.
4. Obtain fresh tissues needed for special studies (cytogenetics, frozen, etc.), as outlined previously.
5. Make cuts parallel to the initial bivalving incision at 2- to 3-cm intervals. Submerge the specimen in a large container of formalin. If the formalin can be refrigerated, color preservation will be enhanced and autolysis slowed.
6. After a few hours or overnight fixation, the remaining sections may be obtained. Two slides should be prepared from all tissue blocks to expedite the mailing of slides to the external review pathologist. The majority of the routine tumor sections should be taken from the periphery of the lesion, showing the following:
   a. Nature of the tumor–kidney junction.
   b. Relationship of the tumor to the renal capsule, particularly in areas of concern for capsular penetration.
   c. Relationship of the tumor to the renal sinus.

TABLE 35-1. Common small blue cell tumors of childhood and diagnostic parameters.

Tumor type	Histology	Immunohistochemistry				EM	Cytogenetics
		NSE	Actin	MIC2	CLA		
Neuroblastoma	Neuropil; ganglionic differentiation Rosettes	+ + +	−	−	−	Neurosecretory granules, processes containing neurofilaments or neurotubules	1p del n-myc amplification
Peripheral neuroectodermal tumor	Rosettes sometimes	+	−	+ +	−	Scant neurosecretory granules, rare processes	t(11;22)
Ewing's sarcoma	Geographic necrosis	±	−	+ +	−	Glycogen lakes	t(11;22)
Rhabdomyosarcoma							
Alveolar	Alveolar-like spaces	±	+ +	±	−	Myofilaments	t(2;13)
Embryonal	Elongated cells	±	+ +	±	−	Myofilaments	11p15
Lymphoblastic lymphoma		−	−	+ +	+	−	Variable
Burkitt's lymphoma		−	−	−	+ +	−	t(8;14)

CLA, common leukocyte antigen; EM, electron microscopy; MIC2, antibody to the protein coded for by the MIC2 gene; NSE, neuron-specific enolase.

d. Areas of the tumor that appear different (e.g., necrosis, hemorrhage). Always indicate the exact site from which each section is taken. This is most easily done by taking Polaroid photographs (see Chapter 3).

7. Carefully section and inspect the normal kidney, particularly adjacent to the tumor. These areas may show microscopic foci of persistent embryonal tissue known as nephrogenic rests, the potential precursor lesion of nephroblastomas.

8. Submit shave sections of the vascular and ureteral margins and, if present, sections of the adrenal gland. The renal vein margin is particularly important.

Using the above guidelines for submission of blocks, histologic evaluation should then provide the specific tumor diagnosis as well as the stage. The staging currently used for pediatric tumors is provided in Table 35-2. The majority of these tumors are stage I at the time of initial resection. The diagnosis of stage II neoplasms depends on the identification of either renal capsular penetration or invasion of the "renal sinus". The renal sinus is the principal portal of exit for tumor cells from the kidney and therefore deserves careful study. The renal sinus is the concave portion of the kidney that contains much of the pelvicalyceal system, and the principal arteries, veins, lymphatics, and nerves that pass through this sinus. It is largely filled with vascularized adipose tissue. The medial border of the sinus is defined by an imaginary plane connecting the most medial portions of the upper and lower poles, termed the *hilar plane*. The renal sinus can be recognized histologically by the fact that the renal cortex lining the sinus lacks a capsule. A thick capsule surrounds the pelvicalyceal structures and continues to cover the medullary pyramids. The distinction between stage I and stage II tumors includes either penetration of the renal capsule or significant invasion of the renal sinus. The criteria for establishing significant invasion have yet to be firmly defined; however, infiltration of vessels and soft tissue of the sinus beyond the hilar plane is considered stage II. Some stage I tumors can distort the renal sinus and protrude beyond the hilar plane with a smoothly encapsulated surface without invading the soft tissue of the renal sinus. Such tumors do not meet the criteria for upstaging, unless they show renal capsular penetration.

TABLE 35-2. Staging of pediatric renal neoplasms (From National Wilms' Tumor Study).

Stage I: Tumor confined to kidney, completely excised
  Intact renal capsule (inflammatory pseudocapsule may be present)
  Infiltrated but not penetrated renal capsule
  Renal sinus not infiltrated beyond hilar plane
  Renal vein contains no tumor (intrarenal vessels may be involved)
  Lymph nodes contain no tumor
  No distant metastases

Stage II: Tumor extends out of the kidney but is completely excised, and there is no evidence of nodal or distant metastases.
  Tumor penetrates renal capsule into perirenal fat
  Tumor capsule biopsied, without diffuse peritoneal spillage
  Tumor infiltrates renal sinus beyond hilar plane
  Tumor in renal vein, removed without cutting across tumor
  Tumor infiltrates adjacent organs or vena cava, but is completely resected

Stage III: Tumor extends outside the kidney
  Tumor incompletely excised
  Surgical margins involved by tumor
  Tumor in lymph nodes
  Tumor thrombus transected
  Peritoneal implants present

Important Issues to Address in Your Report on Pediatric Renal Neoplasms

• What procedure was performed, and what structures/organs are present?
• What type of neoplasm is present? The most common diagnoses in children are Wilms' tumor, clear cell sarcoma, rhabdoid tumor, congenital mesoblastic nephroma, and renal cell carcinoma. If Wilms' tumor, state whether the histology is *favorable* or *unfavorable*. Unfavorable histology is based on the presence of cells with nuclei four times the size of surrounding blastemal cells, or the presence of aberrant mitotic figures. If unfavorable histology (also called *anaplasia*) is present, comment on its extent.
• What is the size of the tumor?
• Are any margins involved?
• Is the renal vein involved by tumor?
• Is renal capsular penetration present?
• Is renal sinus invasion present?

XII   The Central Nervous System

36 Brain and Spinal Cord

Peter C. Burger, M.D.

General Comments

In some respects, pathologic evaluation of specimens from the central nervous system (CNS) is less complicated than evaluation of other organs, because requests for margins and the need for extensive specimen dissections are unusual. On the other hand, CNS specimens are usually small, and care must be taken to preserve the tissue. Do not use all of the tissue by freezing the entire specimen. This is especially true for specimens of the spinal cord. These can be minute, yet major therapeutic decisions often depend on the results of the pathology studies. In all cases, it is essential to keep the clinical and radiological findings in mind when processing specimens from the CNS.

Cytological Preparations

Cytological preparations are essential in the frozen section and permanent section evaluation of all surgically excised brain lesions. These should be prepared in every case for which a frozen section is requested. As illustrated, the preferred procedure is as follows: A minute portion of the fresh specimen is placed on a glass slide and, with considerable pressure, smeared between an opposing slide. The slides are separated and immersed *immediately* in 95% alcohol. Following fixation for 45 to 60 seconds, the preparation is stained and coverslipped.

Needle Biopsy Specimens

Needle biopsy specimens need to be interpreted and handled with special care. The evaluation should begin with cognizance of the clinical and radiographic findings. The chance of making an error is vastly increased when these specimens are studied in a vacuum devoid of clinical or radiographic information.

Begin your examination with the cytological preparation as described above. The remaining fragments of tissue can then be used for a frozen section. Unless you are assured of additional tissue, it is generally wise to freeze only one or two cores at the time of initial examination, holding others in reserve. Throughout the process, review these slides in reference to the radiographic images to ensure that abnormal tissue is obtained and that the findings are consistent with the images. Close contact with the surgeon is extremely important. As is true for biopsies from other body sites, small specimens can be colored with eosin to facilitate identification at the time of embedding and sectioning.

Frozen Sections/Permanent Sections

Freezing must be accomplished as rapidly as possible to minimize the formation of ice crystals. Ice crystals are generally avoidable in certain neoplasms, such as meningiomas, but frequently not in infiltrating gliomas from edema-rich white matter. The recommended procedure is to establish a base of semifrozen mounting medium on a cold chuck. The medium should not be completely frozen, because solidly frozen medium will slowly freeze the tissue and encourage the formation of ice crystals by gradually drawing heat from the small specimen. Therefore, place the specimen on the partially frozen

Press hard, pull apart, and immediately immerse in 95% alcohol.

Small Brain Biopsies for Glial Neoplasms

1. Take a 1 mm core of the specimen and smear it between 2 glass slides. Immediately fix the slides in 95% alcohol, and then stain them for cytologic evaluation.

2. Avoid freezing all of the tissue when a frozen section evaluation is requested. Set a portion of the tissue aside for routine processing, or find out from the surgeon if more tissue will be provided later.

3. When performing a frozen section, freeze the tissue rapidly. Rapid freezing will minimize tissue distortion caused by the formation of ice crystals.

base, and immediately immerse it in liquid nitrogen. After freezing, the specimen can then be covered with additional mounting medium and refrozen. Cut and stain sections by standard methods.

In the case of gliomas, especially the well-differentiated variety, (e.g., astrocytoma and oligodendroglioma), it is extremely important that blocks be available from tissue that is *not* subject to prior frozen section. Prior freezing produces nuclear angulation and hyperchromatism, which can make it difficult to distinguish between gliomas and to distinguish reactive or normal brain from an infiltrating glioma. Unless you are assured of more tissue by the surgeon, use only a portion of the specimen for a frozen section.

Electron Microscopy

To a large extent, immunohistochemistry has replaced electron microscopy as a diagnostic tool; however, in certain instances the latter technique is invaluable. Accordingly, it is appropriate to hold some tissue in reserve in glutaraldehyde (embedding later if necessary) for neoplasms for which classification may be difficult after review of the frozen section. Tissue may also be embedded from encephalitic lesions if viruses are suspected, because no immunohistochemical agents are commercially available for many classes of potential viral pathogens.

Processing of Tissues From Specific Entities

Meningiomas are frequently submitted with a dural attachment and arrive as either a complete en bloc excision or more often, as a series of small fragments. Prognostically significant information relates to histologic features of the lesion as well as the interface of the tumor with surrounding tissues, that is, the brain and the skull. The surface of the mass adjacent to the brain should be sectioned, if identified, particularly if portions of the brain adhere to the surface. At least one section through the base of the tumor on the dura should also be taken.

Decalcified sections of bone are appropriate to evaluate skull invasion.

Schwannomas, commonly either from cranial nerve VIII or the spinal nerve root, are virtually always well differentiated and benign. Therefore, they do not require extensive histologic sampling.

Gliomas are an exceedingly heterogeneous group in terms of their macroscopic and microscopic characteristics. Generally, margins are not an issue and do not, unless specifically stated by the surgeon, affect the treatment of the patient. Fragments of ependymomas, oligodendrogliomas, and astrocytomas, in which little normal brain is recognized, do not need to be sampled in regard to the extent of the disease, although it is prudent to attempt such a localization. In larger en bloc specimens of gliomas, however, a series of marked and recorded sections passing from the tumor into the macroscopically normal brain is appropriate. In the case of malignant gliomas with central necrosis, the most diagnostic tissue is usually found in the cellular rim immediately surrounding the necrotic area. Sections from this area are therefore appropriate. In the case of well-differentiated gliomas (e.g., astrocytoma and oligodendroglioma), the tissue may not appear markedly abnormal, and multiple sections are necessary, particularly from areas in which the white matter is discolored.

Lymphomas are generally recognized during the frozen section process and, in the sporadic form in the nonimmunocompromised patient, they are often suspected on the basis of the neuroimaging features. In this setting, tissue can be reserved frozen for special marker studies (see Chapter 37), although most of the relevant markers for the simple purpose of establishing a clinical diagnosis can be performed on paraffin-embedded sections.

Creutzfeldt-Jakob disease is a rare disorder that is occasionally diagnosed in a cortical biopsy specimen. Although there appears to be only a very small likelihood that pathology personnel will contract Creutzfeldt-Jakob disease from these specimens, caution is appropriate considering the devastating consequences of this disease. Details of this issue are discussed by Brown.[8] Basically, the tissues are fixed in a standard formalin solution for at least 48 hours. The tissues are then placed in a cassette and decontaminated by immersion with periodic agitation in a 95% formic acid solution. The tissue will turn clear. After this, the tissue is placed in formalin again for 1 to 2 days. The tissues can then be treated as any other routine specimen, although some laboratories prefer to hand process them separately. Generally, frozen sections are not recommended on tissues from demented patients.

Important Issues to Address in Your Surgical Pathology Report on Brain and Spinal Cord Biopsies

- What procedure was performed?
- What are the type and grade of the neoplasm? (For glial neoplasms, be sure to document the grading system employed.)
- What is the size of the neoplasm?

XIII   The Hematopoietic and Lymphatic System

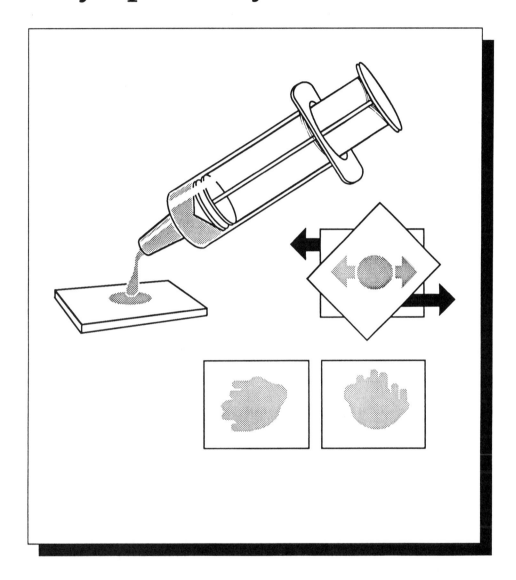

Lymph Nodes

High-quality sections for routine light microscopy are necessary, but not always sufficient, for the interpretation of lymph node biopsies. Immunophenotypic and genetic studies are often required for the diagnosis and classification of a hematopoietic neoplasm. Adequate fixation and timely and appropriate technical handling of lymph nodes are, therefore, even more important than with other specimens.

When lymph nodes are placed in an empty specimen container or in dry gauze, the edges of the specimen dry out, producing a prominent desiccation artifact at the edge of the node. Severe edge artifacts can be introduced into a lymph node even before the specimen reaches the surgical pathology laboratory. Surgeons should therefore be instructed to place resected lymph nodes immediately into a balanced physiologic solution such as Roswell Park Memorial Institute medium (RPMI) 640 or isotonic saline, and to transport lymph nodes immediately to the surgical pathology laboratory. Remember that lymph nodes can also dry out on the cutting table, so proceed quickly and efficiently after removing the specimen from the transport media.

Once the specimen is received, document its size, weight, and shape, and then slice it into uniformly thin 2- to 3-mm sections. Examine the cut surfaces of the node, and ask the following questions: Is the nodal architecture preserved? If the architecture is ablated, is the node grossly nodular, or is the process diffuse? Are any focal lesions present? Is the capsule intact? What is the appearance of the perinodal tissues?

Next, prepare touch imprints by placing the surface of a glass slide against the cut surface of the lymph node. At least five air-dried slides should be prepared, especially in cases of suspected Burkitt's lymphoma, lymphoblastic lymphoma, and myelogenous leukemia. These can be used later for Giemsa stains, oil red O stains, acid phosphatase stains, chloracetate esterase stains, and immunofluorescence for nuclear terminal transferase. Two additional imprints immediately fixed in 95% alcohol should be prepared for possible hematoxylin and eosin (H&E) staining.

Next, tissue should be submitted for light microscopy and, if sufficient tissue is available, for immunohistochemical and genetic studies. Sections for light microscopy should include not only the substance of the node, but also the capsule and perinodal soft tissues. Submit at least one section for fixation in neutral buffered formalin and at least one section in B-5 or an equivalent fixative. The B-5 fixative contains mercuric chloride as well as formaldehyde, and it provides crisp nuclear detail. If a section is submitted in a mercury-based fixative, remember to notify your tissue processing laboratory personnel because these sections require special processing.

The best techniques for submitting fresh tissue for immunophenotyping will depend on your individual laboratory, but in general, a representative section of the node should be snap-frozen in optimal controlled temperature embedding medium for frozen tissue specimens (OCT) for immunohistochemical studies, and a separate 0.5- to 0.7-cm cube should be submitted fresh for flow cytometry. Again, the rapid handling of tissue for these studies is crucial, because delays can result in diffusion artifacts during immunostaining. If tissue will be sent off-site for these analyses, it should not be fro-

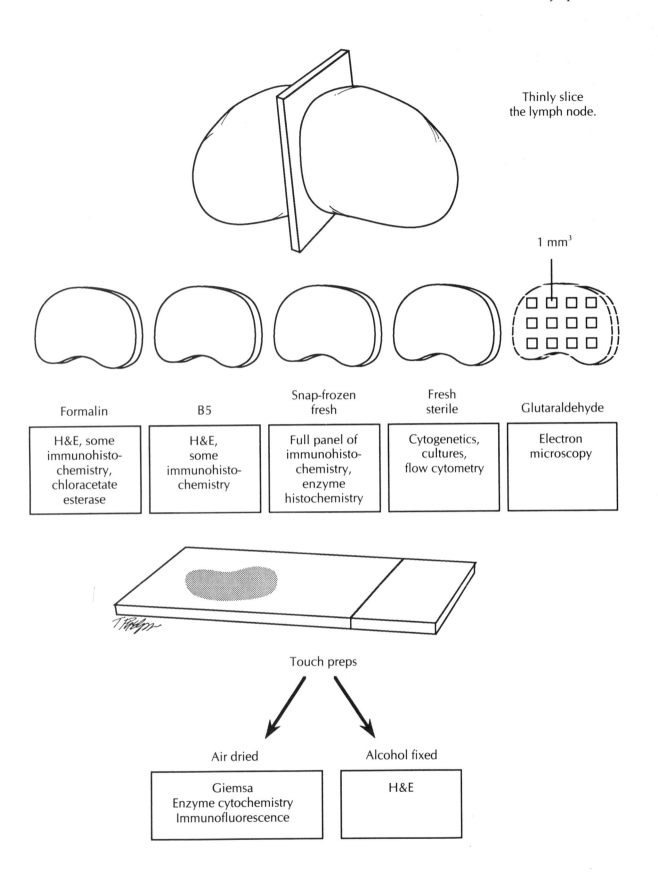

Thinly slice
the lymph node.

1 mm³

Formalin

H&E, some
immunohisto-
chemistry,
chloracetate
esterase

B5

H&E,
some
immunohisto-
chemistry

Snap-frozen
fresh

Full panel of
immunohisto-
chemistry,
enzyme
histochemistry

Fresh
sterile

Cytogenetics,
cultures,
flow cytometry

Glutaraldehyde

Electron
microscopy

Touch preps

Air dried

Giemsa
Enzyme cytochemistry
Immunofluorescence

Alcohol fixed

H&E

zen, but instead it should be kept cool on ice and rapidly transported.

If adequate tissue is available, and it usually is, fresh tissue should also be sent for genetic studies such as gene rearrangements and karyotyping. Submitting this tissue is important because antigen receptor gene rearrangement analysis may be required in those rare cases for which morphology and immunohistochemistry alone cannot establish the diagnosis. Obtain instructions on how to submit these specimens properly from your genetics laboratory.

Finally, if an infection is suspected or granulomas are encountered on a preliminary frozen section evaluation, fresh sterile tissue should be submitted for microbiological studies. If a solid tumor is in the differential diagnosis, then consider placing a small piece of tissue into glutaraldehyde for electron microscopy.

Clearly, the take-home message here is that ''a stitch in time saves nine.'' Even the most challenging hematopoietic neoplasm can be diagnosed if well-fixed tissue for light microscopy and rapidly submitted fresh tissue for special studies are available. Table 37-1 summarizes the type of tissues to be submitted for specific staining methods and other analyses.

Important Issues to Address in Your Surgical Pathology Report on Lymph Nodes

- What procedure was performed, and what structures/organs are present?
- Anatomically, from where were the lymph nodes removed?
- What are the type and grade of the neoplasm?
- What are the number and size of the lymph nodes involved by tumor?

TABLE 37-1. Tissues to submit*

Tissue	Purpose
I. Air-dried touch imprints	Giemsa Enzyme cytochemistry—acid phosphatase, etc. Immunofluorescence for terminal transferase
II. Alcohol-fixed touch imprints	Hematoxylin and eosin
III. Formalin fixed, paraffin embedded	Hematoxylin and eosin Basic immunohistochemistry
IV. B-5 fixed	Hematoxylin and eosin Basic immunohistochemistry
V. Snap-frozen fresh tissue	Detailed immunohistochemistry Enzyme histochemistry

VI. Fresh sterile tissue	Cytogenetics
	    Gene rearrangements
	    Karyotyping
	Microbial cultures
	Flow cytometry

VII. Glutaraldehyde	Electron microscopy

*Modified from Jaffee ES. *Surgical Pathology of the Lymph Nodes and Related Organs.* 2nd ed. Philadelphia, Pa: WB Saunders Co; 1995.

38 Spleen

Three elements are essential for the thorough dissection of the spleen: (1) Be familiar with the patient's clinical history. The dissection of a spleen removed for trauma is very different from the dissection of a spleen removed for a hematopoietic malignancy; (2) Remember that fresh tissue for immunophenotypic and genetic studies may be necessary to classify hematopoietic neoplasms involving the spleen; and (3) Sections of the spleen for histology need to be very thinly sliced and well fixed.

Once resected, the spleen should immediately be brought fresh to the surgical pathology laboratory. The spleen should then be weighed and measured. Next, examine the appearance of the splenic capsule. This step is particularly important in cases of trauma. In particular, document whether the capsule is intact or lacerated, and if it is tense or wrinkled. Next, examine splenic hilum for lymph nodes. If any are found, they should be removed and a representative section of each submitted for histology.

Section the spleen in whichever plane you want, just make sure to section it thinly. Use a long sharp blade to cut the spleen into 2- to 3-mm slices. Examine both sides of each slice for any lesions. Carefully document both the white and red pulp. Expansion of the white pulp gives the cut surface the appearance of white nodules on a red background, while expansion of the red pulp gives the cut surface of the spleen a diffuse red appearance. This step is important because some diseases, such as non-Hodgkin's lymphoma, preferentially involve the white pulp, while others, such as Gaucher's disease, myeloproliferative disorders, and hairy cell leu-

kemia, preferentially involve the red pulp. If nodules are present, count the number of discrete nodules. If the spleen was removed for trauma and if no nodules are found, submit two to four sections of the splenic parenchyma, including a section to demonstrate any parenchymal hemorrhage.

If nodules are present, or if the spleen was removed for a hematopoietic malignancy, then the rest of the approach to the spleen should now follow the approach taken for lymph nodes with suspected hematopoietic malignancies (see Chapter 37). First, prepare touch imprints. Take touch imprints from any discrete nodules. Before preparing these imprints, remove excess blood by blotting the surface of the spleen with a towel. Prepare at least five air-dried and two 95% alcohol-fixed slides.

Next, submit fresh tissue for immunophenotyping. Although the exact techniques vary among laboratories, in general, a representative section should be snap-frozen in optimal controlled temperature embedding medium for frozen tissue specimens (OCT) for immunohistochemical studies, and a separate 0.5- to 0.7-cm tube should be submitted fresh for flow cytometry. Fresh tissue should also be sent for genetic studies such as gene rearrangements and karyotyping, and if clinically indicated, fresh sterile tissue should be submitted for microbiological studies. If multiple types of nodules are present, each type should be separately submitted for these ancillary studies.

Next, tissue should be submitted for light microscopy. Submit thin sections so that they can fix well, and submit at least one section representing each type of lesion seen and one section that includes the splenic capsule. It is not necessary, and in fact not desired, for sections to fill the tissue cassette completely. If multiple small nodules are present, submit two to four representative sections. If both large and small nodules are seen, each must be represented in sampling. If the spleen is enlarged but no lesions are noted, three to four sections are sufficient. As was true for lymph nodes, at least one section should be fixed in B-5 or an equivalent fixative. (If you do submit a section in B-5, remember to notify your tissue processing laboratory because these sections require special processing.) If a storage disease is suspected, tissue should also be fixed in glutaraldehyde for possible electron microscopy.

Important Issues to Address in Your Surgical Pathology Report on Splenectomies

- What procedure was performed, and what structures/organs are present?
- What is the weight of the spleen?
- Is the white pulp architecture normal, more prominent than usual, or obscured (as by a diffuse red pulp infiltrate)?
- In the case of splenic trauma, is the capsule torn, and how much intraparenchymal hemorrhage is present?
- In the case of hematopoietic neoplasm, what type and grade of neoplasm is present, and how many discrete neoplastic nodules are present?

39 Thymus

The thymus, along with the lower pair of parathyroid glands, is derived from the third and fourth pharyngeal pouches. The right and left halves of the gland fuse to form a pyramidal-shaped organ enclosed by a thin fibrous capsule. The thymus has a vital location adjacent to the important organs of the mediastinum. The gland usually sits in the anterosuperior portion of the mediastinum, with the base of the thymus sitting on the pericardium and the upper poles of each lobe extending superiorly into the neck.

Your dissection should start with what is perhaps the most important step in examining the thymus—a careful examination of the surface of the specimen. Is the organ well encapsulated, or is there evidence of invasion into adjacent structures? Are pieces of lung, pericardium, or blood vessels present? Document the degree of encapsulation. Next, weigh the specimen, measure it in all three dimensions, and ink the surfaces of the gland. The gland can then be sectioned at 2- to 3-mm intervals. In infants, the cut surface of the thymus is pink, but by adulthood, much of the parenchyma has been replaced by yellow fat. Describe the cut surface of the gland.

Is it uniform and lobated, cystic or solid? Is there evidence of necrosis or fibrosis? Any grossly identifiable lesions should be measured, and sections should be submitted from each lesion to demonstrate the relationship of the tumor to adjacent structures, to the inked margins, and to any attached tissues. If no grossly identifiable lesions are noted, submit four representative sections for histology. Save the specimen because you may have to go back to it, depending on the patient's clinical history.

Important Issues to Address in Your Surgical Pathology Report on Thymectomies

- What procedure was performed, and what structures/organs are present?
- What are the size and weight of the thymus?
- Is the thymus partially or totally encapsulated?
- What are the type and grade of any neoplasms identified?
- If a tumor is present, does it extend to a margin or into adjacent structures?

40 Bone Marrow

The evaluation of the bone marrow typically includes both a trephine core biopsy and a fluid aspiration. The details of the preparation of these specimens are beyond the scope of this manual; however, you should be familiar with some basics.

Trephine core biopsies are usually 1.0 to 3.0 cm in length and 0.1 to 0.2 cm in diameter. Because of their small size, they generally do not have to be sectioned for further processing. After documenting the size of the biopsy, while it is still fresh, prepare imprints from the biopsy by gently touching the bony fragments to glass slides. These smears should be air dried for later Wright's staining or other special studies such as cytochemical and immunohistochemical analyses. Next, submit the entire core biopsy for processing. The choice of fixatives will depend on your individual institution, but most laboratories like to fix bone marrow biopsies in either Zenker's fixative (for at least 4 hours), buffered formalin (for at least 18 to 24 hours), B-5 (for 4 hours), Bouin's (for 4 to 12 hours), or a mixture of buffered formalin and ethylenediaminetetraacetic acid (EDTA). Once fixed, the specimen can be embedded in either paraffin or plastic. Although paraffin embedding is certainly easier, plastic embedding has the advantage of minimizing artifacts produced by inadequate decalcification.

Usually, approximately 1 cc of liquid is obtained from a bone marrow aspirate. Nine to ten smears should be made *immediately*, before the fluid clots. These smears can be prepared much in the same way as peripheral blood smears are made. To make smears on a coverslip, place a drop on the edge of one coverslip, cover it with another coverslip placed at an angle, and as the drop spreads, pull the two coverslips apart rapidly and smoothly. Alternatively, one drop of the aspirate can be placed at one end of a glass slide and then gently smeared using a pusher coverslip, as illustrated. These smears should be air dried. The remaining aspirate should be placed in an anticoagulant such as EDTA and taken to the hematology laboratory for further processing, which might include iron staining, the preparation of additional smears, and possible electron microscopy. Generally, additional aspirates should be obtained for ancillary studies such as cytogenetics and flow cytometry.

Finally, excess aspirate fluid that has been allowed to clot can be submitted to the laboratory for histologic processing after it has been fixed in formalin.

Important Issues to Address in Your Surgical Pathology Report on the Bone Marrow

- Describe the cellularity, the relative numbers of myeloid and erythroid elements, and their degree of maturation. The marrow biopsy can be used to assess quantitative aspects of maturation, but subtle qualitative aspects are best appreciated on the aspirate.
- Describe the number of megakaryocytes, their arrangement, and any cytologic abnormalities.
- Note the degree and pattern of marrow fibrosis.
- Are there any increases in lymphocytes or plasma cells (include the pattern of infiltration and their cytology)?
- Is an extrinsic tumor present?
- Is the bone itself normal or abnormal?

Two-coverslip technique

Slide and coverslip technique

Bone Marrow Aspirate

1. Two coverslip technique: place a drop on the edge of one coverslip and cover it with another coverslip placed at an angle. Pull the coverslips apart rapidly and smoothly.

2. Slide and coverslip technique: place a drop on the edge of a slide. Position a coverslip at an angle at the edge of the drop and push the coverslip smoothly and rapidly across the slide.

Each of these features should be commented on in the surgical pathology report, although a very brief description can suffice for features that are normal. Where possible, information from both the biopsy, aspirate, and other ancillary studies should be combined to make a definitive diagnosis. In cases for which only a biopsy is available, sometimes only a descriptive diagnosis is given. This practice varies from institution to institution.

XIV   Odds and Ends

41 Common Uncomplicated Specimens

The dissection of tonsils, adenoids, hernia sacs, intervertebral discs, and amputations for gangrene are fairly straightforward, yet a brief discussion of the appropriate handling of these specimens is important for two reasons. First, because these specimens are so frequently encountered, even small mistakes in technique can be magnified over the course of handling numerous specimens. By getting it right the first time, you can avoid developing bad habits that are perpetuated with subsequent dissections. Second, mundane specimens are particularly susceptible to cursory and inattentive examinations. As is true for novel and complex specimens, the prosector should carefully examine the specimen and tailor a dissection that is attuned to the clinical context.

Tonsils and Adenoids

The term *tonsils* usually refers to the palatine tonsils. These are located laterally on each side of the oral cavity as it communicates with the oropharynx. The term *adenoids* refers to the pharyngeal tonsils. These are located along the roof of the nasal cavity as it communicates with the nasopharynx. Even when these two structures are received together in the same specimen container, they can easily be distinguished by their gross appearance. The palatine tonsils are oval-shaped nodules of tissue. They are longer vertically than they are horizontally. Their attached (i.e., lateral) surface is covered by a thick fibrous capsule with adherent soft tissues, while their free (i.e., medial) surface is covered by a tan, glistening mucosa and is somewhat cerebriform in contour, which is due to a longitudinal cleft and stellate crypt openings. The adenoids, on

the other hand, tend to be flat and are frequently fragmented when removed. Their free (mucosal) surfaces are disrupted by deep longitudinal clefts that extend into the underlying lymphoid tissue.

The palatine tonsils are usually removed from both sides of the oropharynx. Subtle changes in the size, shape, and consistency of the tonsils can be appreciated by comparing the two tonsils. For example, enlargement that is due to an infiltrative process may best be appreciated when the enlarged tonsil is compared to the normal tonsil from the opposite side. After the tonsils and adenoids are identified, they should be separately measured and described. Look for exophytic masses, ulcerations, bulky enlargement, and any other gross abnormalities. Bivalve the tonsils and adenoids along the long axis of each, and carefully inspect the cut surface for masses, abscess formation, or other lesions.

Tonsils and adenoids do not always need to be submitted for histologic evaluation. The decision to sample these specimens depends on the patient's clinical history and the gross findings. From our own experience, we have found that these specimens *should* be sampled for histologic evaluation if they meet any of the criteria listed below:

1. The age of the patient is greater than 10 or less than 3 years.
2. The tonsils or adenoids are grossly abnormal.
3. The tonsils or adenoids are greater than 3 cm.
4. There is a size disparity between the two tonsils.
5. Histologic evaluation is requested by the clinician or is indicated by the patient's clinical history.

If any one of the above criteria is met, the tonsils and adenoids should be appropriately sampled for histologic evaluation. One or two representative sections of the tonsils and adenoids are generally sufficient, but certain conditions may require special processing or more extensive sectioning. For example, diffusely enlarged tonsils or adenoids with architectural effacement may suggest involvement by a lymphoproliferative disorder, and these should be processed like a lymph node involved by a lymphoma (see Chapter 37). Sometimes the tonsils are removed in an attempt to find an "occult" primary neoplasm in a patient presenting with metastatic carcinoma to cervical lymph nodes. In this situation, the tonsils should be serially sectioned and submitted in their entirety for histologic evaluation. If the tonsils or adenoids do not meet any of the above criteria, they do not need to be sampled for histologic evaluation. After completing your gross description, place the specimen in formalin and store it for at least 2 weeks.

Hernia Sacs

Hernia sacs are pouches of peritoneum enclosing a hernia. Grossly and microscopically, these are unimpressive specimens. They consist of variable amounts of fat, fibroconnective tissue, and a mesothelial-lined peritoneum. Nonetheless, even hernia sacs attest to the dictum that unexpected but important pathologic findings can be discovered in the most mundane of specimens. Indeed, a wide range of pathologic findings have been documented in routinely resected hernia sacs, ranging from endometriosis to malignant mesothelioma.

Measure and describe the sac, taking note of any areas that appear hemorrhagic or discolored. Palpate the specimen, and document whether or not any nodules are present. Small specimens do not require additional sectioning. Larger tissue fragments should be serially sectioned. Most hernia sacs can be entirely submitted in a single tissue cassette for histologic evaluation. For larger specimens, a single cassette with sections representing all components of the specimen is generally sufficient. More extensive sampling may be necessary when focal lesions are identified or when indicated by the patient's clinical history.

Intervertebral Disk Material

Intervertebral disks typically consist of multiple irregular fragments of fibrous tissue, cartilage, and bone in variable proportions. These fragments are small and generally do not require sectioning. Nonetheless, the prosector's role in handling these is not inconsequential. The appropriate sampling and processing of these specimens largely depends on the prosector's skill at recognizing the various components that are present.

Begin by measuring the specimen. This can be done most efficiently by measuring the aggregate dimensions of the specimen (not the dimensions of each individual piece). Describe the type and appearance of the tissue received. Separate the bone from the soft tissue fragments, and decalcify the pieces of bone so that they can be sectioned by the histology laboratory (see Chapter 2). Keep in mind that these small bone fragments do not require nearly as much time to decalcify as sections from large bone resections. After the bone has been separated, submit the soft tissues for histologic evaluation. Again, if all of the tissue does not easily fit into a single tissue cassette, submit fragments that are representative of the specimen as a whole. Sometimes the patient's clinical history may indicate more extensive sampling, as when metastatic carcinoma is suspected clinically.

Amputations for Gangrene

Admittedly, most amputation specimens are neither small nor anatomically simple. On the other hand, the dissection of amputations for gangrene is straightforward and need not entail an inordinate amount of time and effort. The dissection of these specimens, whether a resection of a digit or an entire limb, should focus on two key questions: What are the nature and extent of the lesion (e.g., ulceration and gangrene)? And what is the underlying pathologic process (e.g., vascular occlusion)? As for all specimens, the patient's clinical history should be clarified before the dissection of an amputation specimen is begun. Clinical and radiographic findings may direct the dissection to the most relevant areas of the specimen.

First, measure the overall dimensions of the

specimen. Make liberal use of anatomic landmarks (e.g., tibial tubercle, lateral tibial malleolus, etc.) when measuring the specimen and describing the location of any lesions. Next, examine the four components of the specimen—the skin, soft tissues, bone, and vasculature. Begin with the skin. Look for loss of hair, skin discoloration, and frank ulceration. Note the location of these findings. Next, evaluate the soft tissues. Section through any ulcers to determine the depth of the ulcer. Do the surrounding soft tissues appear necrotic? Also note whether or not the soft tissues at the surgical margin appear viable. The bone underlying areas of ulceration and necrosis is most likely to reveal pertinent pathology. Specifically, section through the deepest area of any ulcer, and determine if the underlying bone is grossly involved by the inflammatory process. Finally, evaluate the vasculature. For amputations of the lower limbs, occlusive vascular disease can usually be documented by performing a limited dissection of the anterior and posterior tibial arteries. These can be located by sectioning deeply into the anterior and posterior compartments of the calf. A deep transverse incision at midcalf can usually accomplish this. When a complete dissection of a particular vascular tree is indicated, an anatomy text outlining the distribution of the blood supply should be consulted.

Sections should be taken to demonstrate ischemic changes in the skin, necrosis of the soft tissue, inflammation in the underlying bone, occlusive disease of the vascular tree, and viability of the soft tissues at the surgical margin. When sampling the ulcer, include the adjacent epidermis and the underlying subcutaneous tissues. If the zone of ulceration and necrosis appears to extend to the bone, submit a section of the bone immediately underlying the ulcer. Submit cross sections of the major arteries, selectively sampling those regions where the lumen is most stenotic. Finally, submit a transverse section of the neurovascular bundle at the resection margin, along with some skin and soft tissue from this region.

Closing Comments

"But if we are to be in the front lines, then we must make sure that we are better protected in all respects. I am living proof that it can happen to any of us. And no other health care worker should have to go through what I have endured."

Dr. Hacib Aoun
(from "When a House Officer Gets AIDS")[9]

It is our hope that this "hands-on" guide has provided the reader with a logical and concise approach to surgical pathology dissection. Although details of dissection vary from specimen to specimen, we have tried to emphasize some general principles. (1) Understand the patient's clinical history before beginning the dissection; (2) Approach each dissection in a systematic and orderly fashion; (3) Document important findings with complete gross descriptions and specimen photography; (4) Be thorough but selective in sampling tissues for histology; (5) Remember ancillary studies, such as flow cytometry, cytogenetics, hormone receptor analyses and molecular studies, which may require specially processed tissue; and (6) Communicate relevant findings in a complete yet concise manner.

While the routine application of these principles is certainly useful, a purely mechanical approach to surgical pathology is no substitute for compassion and caution. Remember that every specimen comes from a living patient who is anxiously awaiting your diagnosis. Try to imagine that the specimen you are handling came from a close relative. A timely and accurate diagnosis can have a significant positive impact on the patient's mental and physical well-being.

Likewise, a purely mechanical approach to specimen dissection can foster carelessness. Great physicians have lost their lives because they have contracted an infectious disease from a needle stick or knife cut.[9] Once the stick or cut has occurred, you cannot go back and reverse events. *Prevention is the key to your safety.* Wear protective clothing, do not rush, and pay attention to what you are doing! These simple steps may save your life.

References

1. Robbins KT, Medina JE, Wolfe GT, Levine PA, Sessions RB, Pruet CW. Standardizing neck dissection terminology. *Arch Otolaryngol Head Neck Surg.* 1991;117:601–605.
2. Morse D, Steiner RM. Cardiac valve identification atlas and guide. In: Morse D, Steiner RM, Fernandez J, eds. *Guide to Prosthetic Cardiac Valves.* New York, NY: Springer-Verlag, 1985:257.
3. Carey K. Board OKs health reform policy, breast implant protocol. *CAP Today.* 1994;8:26–28.
4. Wigglesworth JS, Singer DB, eds. *Textbook of Fetal and Perinatal Pathology.* Boston, Mass: Blackwell Scientific Publications; 1991.
5. Folberg R, Verdick R, Weingeist TA, Montague PR. The gross examination of eyes removed for choroidal and ciliary body melanomas. *Ophthalmology.* 1986;93:1643–1647.
6. Yamashina M. Follicular neoplasms of the thyroid: total circumferential evaluation of the fibrous capsule. *Am J Surg Pathol.* 1992;16:392–400.
7. Beckwith JB. Renal neoplasms of childhood. In *Diagnostic Surgical Pathology, Second Edition.* SS Sternberg (ed). Raven Press, New York. Chapter 42: 1741–1766, 1994.
8. Brown P. Guidelines for high risk autopsy cases: special precautions for Creutzfeldt-Jakob disease. In: Hutchins GM, ed. *Autopsy Performance and Reporting.* Northfield, Ill: College of American Pathologists; 1990:68–74.
9. Aoun H. When a house officer gets AIDS. *N Engl J Med.* 1989;321:693–696.

Suggested Readings

General Approach to Surgical Pathology Specimens

Association of Directors of Anatomic and Surgical Pathology. Standardization of the surgical pathology report. *Am J Surg Pathol* 1992;16:84–86.

Bell JE, Ironside JW. How to tackle a possible Creutzfeldt-Jakob disease necropsy. *J Clin Pathol*. 1993;46:193–197.

Cooke RA, Stewart B. *Colour Atlas of Anatomical Pathology*. New York, NY: Churchill Livingstone; 1987.

Fazzini E, Weber D, Waldo E. *A Manual for Surgical Pathologists*. Springfield, Ill: Charles C Thomas; 1972.

Geller SA, Gerber MA. Guidelines for high risk autopsy. In: Hutchins GM, ed. *Autopsy Performance and Reporting*. Northfield, Ill: College of American Pathologists; 1995:94–97.

International Union Against Cancer. Hermanek P, Henson DE, Hutter RVP, Sobin LH, eds. *TNM Supplement 1993: A Commentary on Uniform Use*. Berlin: Springer-Verlag; 1993.

International Union Against Cancer. Hermanek P, Sobin LH, eds. *TNM Classification of Malignant Tumours*. 4th ed. (2nd rev.) Berlin: Springer-Verlag; 1992.

International Union Against Cancer. Spiessl B, Beahrs OH, Hermanek P, Hutter RVP, Scheibe O, Sobin LH, Wagner G, eds. *TNM Atlas: Illustrated Guide to the TNM/pTNM Classification of Malignant Tumours*. 3rd ed. (2nd rev.). Berlin: Springer-Verlag; 1992.

Lowe DG, Jeffrey IJM. *Surgical Pathology Techniques*. Philadelphia, PA: BC Decker Inc.; 1990.

Markel SF, Hirsch SD. Synoptic surgical pathology reporting. *Hum Pathol* 1991;22:807–810.

Protection of Laboratory Workers From Infectious Disease Transmitted by Blood, Body Fluids, and Tissue. 2nd ed. NCCLS document M29-T2. Villanova, Pa: National Committee on Clinical Laboratory Standards; 1991.

Richardson JM, Redford LK, Motton H, James R, Porterfield J. Protective garb. *N Engl J Med*. 1988;318:1333. Letter.

Rosai J, members of the Department of Pathology, Memorial Sloan-Kettering Cancer Center. Standardized reporting of surgical pathology diagnoses for the major tumor types: a proposal. *Am J Clin Pathol*. 1993;100:240–255.

Rosai J, Bonfiglio TA, Corson JM, et al. Standardization of the surgical pathology report. *Mod Pathol*. 1992;5:197–199.

Schmidt WA. *Principles and Techniques in Surgical Pathology*. Reading, Mass: Addison-Wesley, 1983.

Scully C, Samaranayake L, Martin M. HIV: answers to common questions on transmission, disinfection and antisepsis in clinical dentistry. *Br Dent J*. 1993;175:175–179.

A Summary of Major Provisions of the Final Rule Implementing the Occupational Safety and Health Administration Bloodborne Pathogens Regulation and Supplemental Information. Northfield, Ill: College of American Pathologists; 1992.

Surgical Pathology/Cytopathology Quality Assurance Manual. Northfield, Ill: College of American Pathologists; 1993.

Teloh HA. *Methods in Surgical Pathology*. Springfield, Ill: Charles C Thomas; 1957.

Travers H, Davey D, Cleary K, Tazelaar H, Minielly J, eds. *Quality Improvement Manual in Anatomic Pathology*. Northfield, Ill: College of American Pathologists; 1993.

Laboratory Techniques

Culling CFA. *Handbook of Histopathological and Histochemical Techniques*. 3rd ed. Boston, Mass: Butterworths & Co, Ltd; 1974.

Dawson PJ, Deckys MC. Rapid (same day) processing of biopsies using Carnoy's fixative. *Am J Surg Pathol*. 1987;11:82.

Greer CE, Peterson SL, Kiviat NB, Manos MM. PCR amplification from paraffin-embedded tissues. *Am J Clin Pathol*. 1991;95:117–124.

Hopwood D. Fixation and fixatives. In: Bancroft JD, Stevens A, eds. *Theory and Practice of Histological Techniques*. New York, NY: Churchill Livingstone; 1977:16–28.

Kelley DB, Abt AB. An improved method for mounting frozen-section specimens. *Am J Surg Pathol*. 1990;14:186–187.

Kok LP, Boon ME, Suurmeijer AJH. Major improvement in microscopic-image quality of cryostat sections. Combining freezing and microwave-stimulated fixation. *Am J Clin Pathol*. 1987;88:620–623.

Luna LG, ed. *Manual of Histologic Staining Methods of the Armed Forces Institute of Pathology*, 3rd ed. New York, NY: McGraw-Hill Book Co; 1968.

Naish SJ, Boenisch T, Farmilo AJ, Stead RH, eds. *Handbook. Immunochemical Staining Methods*. Carpinteria, Calif: DAKO Corp; 1989.

Page DL, Nolen C, Womack JL. Histologic technique. *Am J Surg Pathol*. 1989;13:1072. Letter.

Pearse AGE. *Histochemistry. Theoretical and Applied*. 2nd ed. Boston, Mass: Little, Brown, and Co; 1960.

Radivoyevitch MA. Stamping method for frozen section. *Am J Surg Pathol*. 1989;13:244–245.

Rogers C, Klatt EC, Chandrasoma P. Accuracy of frozen-section diagnosis in a teaching hospital. *Arch Pathol Lab Med*. 1987;111:514–517.

Sheehan DC, Hrapchak BB. Fixation. In: Sheehan DC, Hrapchak, BB, eds. *Theory and Practice of Histotechnology*. 2nd ed. St Louis, Mo: CV Mosby Co; 1980;40–58.

SooHoo W, Ruebner B, Vogt P, Wiese D. Orientation of small, flat frozen-section specimens. *Am J Surg Pathol*. 1988;12:573–574.

Start RD, Cross SS, Smith JHF. Assessment of specimen fixation in a surgical pathology service. *J Clin Pathol*. 1992;45:546–547.

Therkildsen MH, Pilgaard J. Microwave-assisted frozen section diagnosis: a comparison between conventional cryostat technique and the combination of freezing and microwave-stimulated fixation. *Acta Pathol Microbiol Immunol Scand*. 1990;98:200–202.

Woosley JT. Improved histology from inadequately fixed paraffin-embedded biopsy specimens. *Am J Surg Pathol*. 1989;13:246–247.

Wright JR Jr. The development of the frozen section technique, the evolution of surgical biopsy, and the origins of surgical pathology. *Bull Hist Med*. 1985; 59:295–326.

Photography

Burgess CA. Gross specimen photography—a survey of lighting and background techniques. *Med Biol Illustr*. 1975;25:159–166.

Cutignola L, Bullough PG. Photographic reproduction of anatomic specimens using ultraviolet illumination. *Am J Surg Pathol*. 1991;15:1096–1099.

Haberlin C. Specimen photography. In: Hansell P, ed. *A Guide to Medical Photography*. London: MTP Press; 1979:77–97.

Vetter JP. The color presentation and photography of gross specimens. *J Audiovis Med*. 1983;6:7–12.

Vetter JP. The color photography of gross specimens. *J Coll Am Pathologist*. 1984;3:155–161.

White W. *Photomacrography, an Introduction*. Boston, Mass: Butterworth Publications; 1987:97–133.

William AR. Closeup photography and photomicrography. In: Morton R, ed. *Photography for the Scientist*. London: London Academic Press; 1984:355–391.

Head and Neck—General

Barnes L, Johnson JT. Pathologic and clinical considerations in the evaluation of major head and neck specimens resected for cancer. *Part I. Pathol Annu*. 1986;21:173–250.

Batsakis JG. *Tumors of the Head and Neck: Clinical and Pathological Considerations*. 2nd ed. Baltimore, Md: Williams & Wilkins; 1979.

Gnepp DR, ed. *Contemporary Issues in Surgical Pathology: Pathology of the Head and Neck*. New York, NY: Churchill Livingstone; 1988.

Larynx

Harwood AR. Cancer of the larynx. *J Otolaryngol*. 1982;11:2–21.

Hollinger LD, Miller AW. A specimen mount for small laryngeal biopsies. *Laryngoscope*. 1982;92:524–526.

Kashima HK. The characteristics of laryngeal cancer correlating with cervical lymph node metastasis (analysis based on 40 total organ sections). *Can J Otolaryngol*. 1975;4:893–902.

Kirchner JA, Carter D. The larynx. In: Sternberg SS, ed. *Diagnostic Surgical Pathology*. New York, NY: Raven Press; 1994:893–916.

Levendag PC, Veeze-Kuijpers B, Knegt PPM, et al. Cancer of the supraglottic larynx with neck node metastasis treated by radiation therapy only: the revised 1987 URIC classification system as prognostic indicator. *Acta Oncol* 1990;29:603–609.

McGavran MH, Bauer WC, Ogura JH. The incidence of cervical lymph node metastases from epidermoid carcinoma of the larynx and their relationship to certain characteristics of the primary tumor. *Cancer* 1961;14:55–66.

Olofsson J. Growth and spread of laryngeal carcinoma. *Can J Otolaryngol*. 3:1974;446–459.

Vermund H. Role of radiotherapy in cancer of the

larynx as related to the TNM system of staging: a review. *Cancer*. 1970;25:485–504.

Salivary Glands

Ellis GL, Auclair PL, Gnepp DR, eds. *Surgical Pathology of the Salivary Glands*. Philadelphia, Pa: WB Saunders Co; 1991.

Radical Neck Dissection

Merlano M, Vittale V, Rosso R, et al. Treatment of advanced squamous-cell carcinoma of the head and neck with alternating chemotherapy and radiotherapy. *N Engl J Med*. 1992;327:1115–1121.

Robbins KT, Medina JE, Wolfe GT, Levine PA, Sessions RB, Pruet CW. Standardizing neck dissection terminology. *Arch Otolaryngol Head Neck Surg*. 1991;117:601–605.

Vikram B, Strong EW, Shah J, Spiro RH. Elective postoperative radiation therapy in stages III and IV epidermoid carcinoma of the head and neck. *Am J Surg*. 1980;140:580–584.

Digestive System—General

Appelman HD, ed. *Contemporary Issues in Surgical Pathology: Pathology of the Esophagus, Stomach, and Duodenum*. New York, NY: Churchill Livingstone; 1984.

Haggitt RC. Handling of gastrointestinal biopsies in the surgical pathology laboratory. *Lab Med*. 1982;13:272–278.

Esophagus

Ming S-C. *Tumors of the Esophagus and Stomach*. Washington, DC: Armed Forces Institute of Pathology; 1973.

Stomach

Japanese Research Society for Gastric Cancer. The general rules for the gastric study in surgery and pathology. Part I. Clinical classification. *Jpn J Surg*. 1981;11:127–139.

Rotterdam H, Enterline HT, *Pathology of the Stomach and Duodenum*. New York, NY: Springer-Verlag, 1989.

Non-Neoplastic Intestinal Disease

Ming SC, Goldman H, eds. *Pathology of the Gastrointestinal Tract*. Philadelphia, Pa: WB Saunders; 1992.

Norris HT, ed. *Pathology of the Colon, Small Intestine, and Anus*. New York, NY: Churchill and Livingstone; 1983.

Neoplastic Intestinal Disease

Henson DE, Hutter RVP, Sobin LH, Bowman HE. Protocol for the examination of specimens removed from patients with colorectal cancer. *Arch Pathol Lab Med*. 1994;118:122–125.

Hermanek P, Giedl J, Dworak O. Two programmes for examination of regional lymph nodes in colorectal carcinoma with regard to the new pN classification. *Pathol Res Pract* 1989;185:867–873.

Qizilbash AH. Pathologic studies in colorectal cancer: a guide to the surgical pathology examination of colorectal specimens and review of features of prognostic significance. *Pathol Annu*. 1982;17:1–46.

Zarbo RJ. Interinstitutional assessment of colorectal carcinoma surgical pathology report adequacy: a College of American Pathologists Q-probes study of practice patterns from 532 laboratories and 15,940 reports. *Arch Pathol Lab Med*. 1992;116:1113–1119.

Appendix

Gray GF Jr, Wackym PA. Surgical pathology of the vermiform appendix. *Pathol Annu*. 1986;21:111–144.

Liver

Arias IM, Popper H, Shachter D, Shafritz DA. *The Liver: Biology and Pathobiology*. New York: Raven Press; 1982.

Elias H, Sherrick JC. *Morphology of the Liver*. New York, NY: Academic Press; 1969.

Sherlock S. *Diseases of the Liver and Biliary System*. Philadelphia, Pa: FA Davis Co; 1968.

Gallbladder

Albores-Saavedra J, Henson DE. *Atlas of Tumor Pathology: Tumors of the Gallbladder and Extrahepatic Bile Ducts*. Washington, DC: Armed Forces Institute of Pathology; 1986.

Pancreas

Cruickshank AH. *Pathology of the Pancreas*. Berlin: Springer-Verlag; 1986.

Cubilla AL, Fitzgerald PJ. *Atlas of Tumor Pathology: Tumors of the Exocrine Pancreas*. Washington, DC: Armed Forces Institute of Pathology; 1984.

Klöppel G, Heitz PU, eds. *Pancreatic Pathology*. Edinburgh: Churchill Livingstone; 1984.

Heart Valves and Vessels

Hackel DB. Anatomy and pathology of the cardiac conducting system. In: Edwards JE, ed. *The Heart*. Baltimore, Md: Williams & Wilkins; 1974:232–47.

Morse D, Steiner RM. Cardiac valve identification atlas and guide. In: Morse D, Steiner RM, Fernandez J, eds. *Guide to Prosthetic Cardiac Valves*. New York, NY: Springer-Verlag; 1985.

Schoen FJ, Sutton MSJ. Contemporary issues in the pathology of valvular heart disease. *Hum Pathol*. 1987;18:568–576.

Schoen FJ. Symposium on cardiovascular pathology, part II. Surgical pathology of removed natural and prosthetic heart valves. *Hum Pathol*. 1987;18:558–567.

Silver MD. *Cardiovascular Pathology*. New York, NY: Churchill Livingstone, 1983.

Virmani R, Atkinson J, Fenoglio JJ. *Cardiovascular Pathology*. Philadelphia, Pa: WB Saunders; 1991.

Lungs

Association of Directors of Anatomic and Surgical Pathology. Recommendations for the reporting of resected primary lung carcinomas. Mod Pathol 8: 796–798, 1995.

Carter D. Pathologic examination of major pulmonary specimens resected for neoplastic disease. *Pathol Annu*. 1983;18:315–332.

Churg A. An inflation procedure for open lung biopsies. *Am J Surg Pathol*. 1983;7:69–71.

Colby TV, Koss M, Travis WD. *Atlas of Tumors of the Lower Respiratory Tract*. 3rd Series. Washington, DC: Armed Forces Institute of Pathology; 1995.

Dail DH, Hammar SP, eds. *Pulmonary Pathology*. 2nd ed. New York, NY: Springer-Verlag; 1994.

Halbower AC, Mason RJ, Abman SH, Tuder RM. Agarose infiltration improves morphology of cryostat sections of lung. *Lab Invest*. 1994;71:149–153.

Katzenstein A-LA, Askin FB. *Surgical Pathology of Non-neoplastic Lung Disease*. 2nd ed. Philadelphia, Pa: WB Saunders; 1990.

Mark EJ. The second diagnosis: the role of the pathologist in identifying pneumoconioses in lungs excised for tumor. *Hum Pathol* 1981;12:585–587.

Naruke T, Suemasu K, Ishikawa S. Lymph node mapping and curability at various levels of metastasis in resected lung cancer. *J Thorac Cardiovasc Surg*. 1978;76:832–839.

Thurlbeck WM, ed. *Pathology of the Lung*, New York, NY: Thieme Medical Publishers Inc; 1988.

Bone

Dahlin DC. *Bone Tumors: General Aspects and Data on 6,221 Cases*. 3rd ed. Springfield, Ill: Charles C Thomas; 1978.

Fechner RE, Mills SE. *Atlas of Tumor Pathology: Tumors of the Bone and Joints*. 3rd series, fascicle 8. Washington, DC: Armed Forces Institute of Pathology; 1993.

Huvos AG. *Bone Tumors: Diagnosis, Treatment, and Prognosis*. Philadelphia, Pa: WB Saunders Co: 1991.

Vincic L, Weston S, Riddell RH. Bone core biopsies: plastic or paraffin? *Am J Surg Pathol*. 1989;13:329–334.

Soft Tissue, Nerves, and Muscle

Anthony DC, Crain BJ. Practical topics in neuropathology: nerve biopsy. *Arch Pathol Lab Med*. 1996; 120:26–34.

Carpenter S, Karpati G. *Pathology of Skeletal Muscle*. New York, NY: Churchill Livingstone; 1984.

Dabowitz V. *Muscle Biopsy: A Practical Approach*. 2nd ed. Philadelphia, Pa: Baillière Tindall, 1985.

de la Monte SM. Postmortem evaluation of neuromuscular diseases. In: Hutchins GM, ed. *Autopsy. Performance and Reporting*. Northfield, Ill: College of American Pathologists; 1990:99–105.

Enzinger FM, Weiss SW. *Soft Tissue Tumors*. 3rd ed. St Louis, Mo: CV Mosby Co; 1994.

Pearl G, Ghatak N. Practical topics in neuropathology: muscle biopsy. *Arch Pathol Lab Med*. In press.

Skin

Ackerman AB. *Pathology of Malignant Melanoma*. New York, NY: Masson Publishing USA, Inc; 1981.

Elder DE, Murphy GF. *Atlas of Tumor Pathology: Melanocytic Tumors of the Skin*. 3rd series, fascicle 2. Washington, DC: Armed Forces Institute of Pathology; 1991.

Holmes EC, Clark W. Morton DL, Eilber FR, Bochow AJ. Regional lymph node metastases and the level of invasion of primary melanoma. *Cancer* 1976;37: 199–201.

Mondragon G, Nygaard F. Routine and special procedures for processing biopsy specimens for lesions suspected to be malignant melanomas. *Am J Dermatopathol*. 1981;3:265–272.

Murphy GF, Elder DE. *Atlas of Tumor Pathology: Nonmelanocytic Tumors of the Skin*. 3rd series, fascicle 1. Washington, DC: Armed Forces Institute of Pathology; 1991.

White CR Jr. Laboratory handling of skin biopsy specimens. *Lab Med*. 1982;13:211–217.

Breast

Association of Directors of Anatomic and Surgical Pathology. Immediate management of mammographically detected breast lesions. *Am J Surg Pathol.* 1993;17(8):850–851.

Azzopardi JG, Ahmed A, Millis RR. Problems in breast pathology. In: Bennington JL, ed. *Major Problems in Pathology.* Philadelphia, Pa: WB Saunders Co; 1979;2:1.

Carey K. Board OKs health reform policy, breast implant protocol. *CAP Today.* 1994;8:26–28.

Murad TM. What to expect from the pathology report concerning breast tumors. *Ala J Med Sci.* 1975;12: 222–224.

National Cancer Institute. Standardized management of breast specimens. *Am J Clin Pathol.* 1978;60:789–798.

Schnitt SJ, Connolly JL. Processing and evaluation of breast excision specimens: a clinically oriented approach. *Am J Clin Pathol.* 1992;98:125–137.

Gynecologic—General

Gompel C, Silverberg SG, eds. *Pathology in Gynecology and Obstetrics.* 4th ed. Philadelphia, Pa: JB Lippincott; 1994.

Mattingly RF, Thompson JD, eds. *TeLinde's Operative Gynecology.* 6th ed. Philadelphia, Pa: JB Lippincott; 1985.

Nichols DH, ed. *Gynecologic and Obstetric Surgery.* St Louis, Mo: CV Mosby; 1993.

Robboy SJ, Bentley RC, Krigman H, Silverberg SG, Norris HJ, Zaino RJ. Synoptic reports in gynecologic pathology. *Int J Gynecol Pathol.* 1994;13:161–174.

Robboy SJ, Kraus FT, Kurman RJ. Gross description, processing, and reporting of gynecologic and obstetric specimens. In: Kurman RJ, ed. *Blausteins Pathology of the Female Genital Tract.* 4th ed. New York, NY: Springer-Verlag; 1994.

Scully RE, Bonfiglio TA, Kurman RJ, Silverberg SG, Wilkinson EJ. *Histologic Typing of Female Genital Tract Tumors.* 2nd ed. Berlin: Springer-Verlag; 1994.

Vulva, Uterus, Cervix, and Vagina

Fu YS, Reagan JW. *Pathology of the Uterine Cervix, Vagina, and Vulva.* Philadelphia, Pa: WB Saunders, 1989;21.

Kurman RJ, Norris HJ, Wilkinson E. *Atlas of Tumor Pathology: Tumors of the Cervix, Vagina, and Vulva.* 3rd series, fascicle 4. Washington, DC: Armed Forces Institute of Pathology; 1992.

Mazur MT, Kurman RJ. *Diagnosis of Endometrial Biopsies and Curettings.* New York, NY: Springer-Verlag; 1994.

Silverberg SG, Kurman RJ. *Atlas of Tumor Pathology: Tumors of the Uterine Corpus and Gestational Trophoblastic Disease.* 3rd series, fascicle 3. Washington, DC: Armed Forces Institute of Pathology; 1992.

Wilkinson EJ, ed. *Contemporary Issues in Surgical Pathology. Pathology of the Vulva and Vagina.* New York, NY: Churchill Livingstone; 1987;9.

Wright TC, Gagnon S, Richart RM, Ferenczy A. Treatment of cervical intraepithelial neoplasia using the loop electro-surgical excision procedure. *Obstet Gynecol.* 1992;79:173–178.

Ovary and Fallopian Tube

Scully RE. Tumors of the ovary and maldeveloped gonads. In *Atlas of Tumor Pathology.* Fascicle 16, 2nd series. Washington, DC: Armed Forces Institute of Pathology; 1979.

Scully RE, Henson DE, Nielsen M, Ruby SG. Practice protocol for the examination of specimens removed from patients with ovarian tumors. A basis for checklists. *Arch Pathol Lab Med.* 1995; 119:1012–1022.

Woodruff JD, Pauerstein CJ. *The Fallopian Tube: Structure, Function, Pathology and Management.* Baltimore, Md: Williams & Wilkins; 1969.

Young RH, Clement PB, Scully RE. The ovary and the fallopian tube and broad ligament. In: Sternberg SS, ed. *Diagnostic Surgical Pathology.* 2nd ed. New York, NY: Raven Press; 1994; chaps 53, 54.

Products of Conception and Placentas

Benirschke K, Kaufmann P. *Pathology of the Human Placenta.* 2nd ed. New York, NY: Springer-Verlag; 1990.

Driscoll SG, Langston C. College of American Pathologists conference XIX on the examination of the placenta: report of the working group on methods for placental examination. *Arch Pathol Lab Med.* 1991;115:704–708.

Keeling JW, ed. *Fetal and Neonatal Pathology.* London: Springer-Verlag; 1987.

Naeye R. Functionally important disorders of the placenta, umbilical cord, and fetal membranes. *Hum Pathol.* 1987;18:680–691.

Reed GB, Claireaux AE, Bain AD, eds. *Diseases of the Fetus and Newborn: Pathology, radiology and genetics.* St Louis, Mo: CV Mosby; 1989.

Szulman AE. Examination of the early conceptus. *Arch Pathol Lab Med* 1991;115:696–700.

Wigglesworth JS, Singer DB, eds. *Textbook of Fetal and Perinatal Pathology.* Boston, Mass: Blackwell Scientific Publications; 1991.

Penis

Cubilla AL, Barreto J, Caballero C, Ayala G, Riveros M. Pathologic features of epidermoid carcinoma of the penis: a prospective study of 66 cases. *Am J Surg Pathol*. 1993;17:753–763.

Mostofi FK, Price EB. *Tumors of the Male Genital System*. Washington, DC: Armed Forces Institute of Pathology; 1973.

Prostate

Bova GS, Fox WM III, Epstein JI. Methods of radical prostatectomy specimen processing: a novel technique for harvesting fresh prostate cancer tissue and review of processing techniques. *Mod Pathol*. 1993;6:201–207.

Epstein JI. Evaluation of radical prostatectomy capsular margins of resection: the significance of margins designated as negative, closely approaching, and positive. *Am J Surg Pathol*. 1990;14:626–632.

Epstein JI. Evaluation of radical prostatectomy specimens: therapeutic and prognostic implications. *Pathol Annu*. 1991;26:159–210.

Hall GS, Kramer CE, Epstein JI. Evaluation of radical prostatectomy specimens: a comparative analysis of sampling methods. *Am J Surg Pathol*. 1992;16:315–324.

Henson DE, Hutter RVP, Farrow G. Practice protocol for the examination of specimens removed from patients with carcinoma of the prostate gland. *Arch Pathol Lab Med*. 1994;118:779–783.

Moore GH, Lawshe B, Murphy J. Diagnosis of adenocarcinoma in transurethral resectates of the prostate gland. *Am J Surg Pathol*. 1986;10:165–169.

Mostofi FK. Prostate sampling. *Am J Surg Pathol*. 1986;10:175. Letter.

Murphy WM, Dean PJ, Brasfield JA, Tatum L. Incidental carcinoma of the prostate: how much sampling is adequate? *Am J Surg Pathol*. 1986;10:170–174.

Randall A. *Surgical Pathology of Prostatic Obstructions*. Baltimore, Md: Williams & Wilkin; 1931.

Schmid H-P, McNeal JE. An abbreviated standard procedure for accurate tumor volume estimation in prostate cancer. *Am J Surg Pathol*. 1992;16:184–191.

Testis

Borski AA. Diagnosis, staging and natural history of testicular tumors. *Cancer*. 1973;32:1202–1205.

Collins DH, Pugh RCB. *The Pathology of Testicular Tumors*. Edinburgh: E&S Livingstone Ltd; 1964.

Pugh RCB, ed. *Pathology of the Testis*. Oxford, UK: Blackwell Scientific Publications; 1976.

Talerman A, Roth LM, eds. *Contemporary Issues in Surgical Pathology: Pathology of the Testis and Its Adnexa*. New York, NY: Churchill Livingstone; 1986.

Kidney

Holland JM. Cancer of the kidney: natural history and staging. *Cancer*. 1973;32:1030–1042.

Murphy WM, Beckwith JB, Farrow GM. *Atlas of Tumor Pathology: Tumors of the Kidney, Bladder, and Related Structures*. 3rd series, fascicle 11. Washington, DC: Armed Forces Institute of Pathology; 1994.

Bladder

Friedell GH, Parija GC, Nagy GK, Soto EA. The pathology of human bladder cancer. *Cancer*. 1980;45:1823–1831.

Murphy WM, Beckwith JB, Farrow GM. *Atlas of Tumor Pathology: Tumors of the Kidney, Bladder, and Related Structures*. 3rd series, fascicle 11. Washington, DC: Armed Forces Institute of Pathology; 1994.

Skinner DG. Current state of classification and staging of bladder cancer. *Cancer Res*. 1977;37:2838–2842.

Young RH, ed. *Contemporary Issues in Surgical Pathology: Pathology of the Urinary Bladder*. New York, NY: Churchill Livingstone; 1989.

Eye

Apple DJ, Rabb MF. *Ocular Pathology: Clinical Applications and Self-Assessment*. St Louis, Mo: Mosby-Year Book; 1991:1–13.

Beck K, Jensen OA. *External Ocular Tumors. Textbook and Atlas*. Philadelphia, Pa: WB Saunders Co; 1978.

Doxanas MT, Green WR, Iliff CE. Factors in the successful surgical management of basal cell carcinoma of the eyelids. *Am J Ophthalmol*. 1981;91:726–736.

Duane T. *Clinical Ophthalmology*. New York, NY: Harper & Row Publishers Inc; 1976.

Engel H, de la Cruz ZC, Green WR, Michels RG. Cytopreparatory techniques for eye fluid specimens obtained by vitrectomy. *Acta Cytologica*. 1982;26:551–560.

Folberg R, Verdick R, Weingeist TA, Montague PR. The gross examination of eyes removed for choroidal and ciliary body melanomas. *Ophthalmology*. 1986;93:1643–1647.

Hogan MJ, Zimmerman LE. *Ophthalmic Pathology. An Atlas and Textbook*. 2nd ed. Philadelphia, Pa: WB Saunders, 1962.

Luna LG. *Manual of Histologic Staining Methods of the Armed Forces Institute of Pathology*. New York, NY: McGraw-Hill Book Co; 1968:53–54.

Menocal NG, Ventura DB, Yanoff M. Eye techniques: routine processing of ophthalmic tissue for light microscopy. In: Sheehan DC, Hrapchak BB, eds. *Theory and Practice of Histotechnology*. 2nd ed. St Louis, Mo: CV Mosby, 1980:285–291.

Shields JA, Shields CL, Ehya H, Eagle RC Jr, De Potter P. Fine-needle aspiration biopsy of suspected intraocular tumors. *Ophthalmology*. 1993;100:1677–1684.

Spencer WH, ed. *Ophthalmic Pathology: An Atlas and Textbook*. 3rd ed. Philadelphia, Pa: WB Saunders, 1985.

Torczynski E. Preparation of ocular specimens for histopathologic examination. *Ophthalmology*. 1981;88:1367–1371.

Yanoff M, Fine B. *Ocular Pathology. A Text and Atlas*. New York, NY: Harper & Row Publishers Inc; 1975.

Thyroid

LiVolsi VA. *Surgical Pathology of the Thyroid*. Philadelphia, Pa: WB Saunders Co; 1990.

Rosai J, Carcangiu ML, DeLellis RA. *Atlas of Tumor Pathology: Tumors of the Thyroid Gland*, 3rd series, fascicle 5. Washington DC: Armed Forces Institute of Pathology; 1992.

Yamashina M. Follicular neoplasms of the thyroid: total circumferential evaluation of the fibrous capsule. *Am J Surg Pathol*. 1992;16:392–400.

Parathyroid Glands

DeLellis RA. *Atlas of Tumor Pathology: Tumors of the Parathyroid Gland*, 3rd series, fascicle 6. Washington, DC: Armed Forces Institute of Pathology; 1993.

Geelhoed GW, Silverberg SG. Intraoperative imprints for the identification of parathyroid tissue. *Surgery*. 1984;96:1124–1131.

Grimelius L, Åkerström, G, Johansson H, Bergström R. Anatomy and histopathology of human parathyroid glands. *Pathol Annu*. 1981;16:1–24.

LiVolsi VA, Hamilton R. Intraoperative assessment of parathyroid gland pathology: a common view from the surgeon and the pathologist. *Am J Clin Pathol*. 1994;102:365–373.

Adrenal Glands

Lack EE, ed. *Contemporary Issues in Surgical Pathology: Pathology of the Adrenal Glands*. New York, NY: Churchill Livingstone; 1990.

Neville AM, O'Hare MJ. *The Human Adrenal Cortex*. New York, NY: Springer-Verlag; 1982.

Page DL, DeLellis RA, Hough AJ Jr. *Atlas of Tumor Pathology: Tumors of the Adrenal*. 2nd series, fascicle 23. Washington, DC: Armed Forces Institute of Pathology; 1985.

Brain and Spinal Cord

Bell JE, Ironside JW. How to tackle a possible Creutzfeldt-Jakob disease necropsy. *J Clin Pathol*. 1993;46:193–197.

Brown P. Guidelines for high risk autopsy cases: special precautions for Creutzfeldt-Jakob disease. In: Hutchins GM, ed. *Autopsy Performance and Reporting*. Northfield, Ill: College of American Pathologists; 1990;68–74.

Burger PC, Scheithauer BW. *Atlas of Tumor Pathology: Tumors of the Central Nervous System*, 3rd series, fascicle 10. Washington, DC: Armed Forces Institute of Pathology; 1994.

Burger PC, Scheithauer BW, Vogel SF. *Surgical Pathology of the Nervous System and Its Coverings*. New York, NY: Churchill Livingstone; 1991.

Scheithauer BW. Surgical pathology of the pituitary: the adenomas. *Pathol Annu*. 1984;19:317–374.

Lymph Nodes

Crowley KS. Lymph node biopsy. *Pathology*. 1983;15:137–138.

Durkin K, Haagensen CD. An improved technique for the study of lymph nodes in surgical specimens. *Ann Surg*. 1980;191:419–429.

Jaffee ES. *Surgical Pathology of the Lymph Nodes and Related Organs*, 2nd ed. Philadelphia, Pa: WB Saunders Co; 1995.

Mufarrij A, Valensi QJ. A method for the dissection of lymph node specimens (anatomic method). *Am J Surg Pathol*. 1981;5:497–500.

Spleen

Burke JS. Surgical pathology of the spleen: an approach to the differential diagnosis of splenic lymphomas and leukemias. Part 1. Diseases of the white pulp. *Am J Surg Pathol*. 1981;5:551–563.

Burke JS. Surgical pathology of the spleen: an approach to the differential diagnosis of splenic lymphomas and leukemias. Part II. Diseases of the red pulp. *Am J Surg Pathol*. 1981;5:681–694.

Thymus

Nezelof C. Thymic pathology in primary and secondary immunodeficiencies. *Histopathology*. 1992;21:499–511.

Rosai J, Levine GD. *Tumors of the Thymus*. 2nd series, fascicle 13. Washington, DC: Armed Forces Institute of Pathology; 1976.

Bone Marrow

Arber DA, Rainer P, Helbert B, Rappaport ES. Agar processing of bone marrow aspirate material. *Lab Med*. 1992;23:479–484.

Brunning RD, McKenna RW. *Atlas of Tumor Pathology: Tumors of the Bone Marrow*. 3rd series, fascicle 9. Washington, DC: Armed Forces Institute of Pathology; 1994.

Knowles DM, ed. *Neoplastic Hematopathology*. Baltimore, Md: Williams & Wilkins; 1992.

Pediatric Tumors

Coffin CM, Dehner LP. Soft tissue neoplasms in childhood: a clinicopathologic overview. In: Finegold M, Bennington JL, eds. *Pathology of Neoplasia in Children and Adolescents*. Philadelphia, Pa: WB Saunders Co; 1986.

Helwig EB. Malignant melanoma in children. In: *Neoplasms of the Skin and Malignant Melanoma*. Proceedings of the 20th Annual Clinical Conferences on Cancer, Houston, Tex. Chicago, Ill: Year Book Medical Publishers, Inc; 1975:11–26.

Pochedly C, Miller D, Finklestein JZ. *Wilms' Tumor*. New York, NY: John Wiley & Sons; 1976.